REVERSING NEUROPATHY: THE F.R.E.E.D.O.M. METHOD

REVERSING NEUROPATHY: THE F.R.E.E.D.O.M. METHOD

DR. JASON TRIPP DC

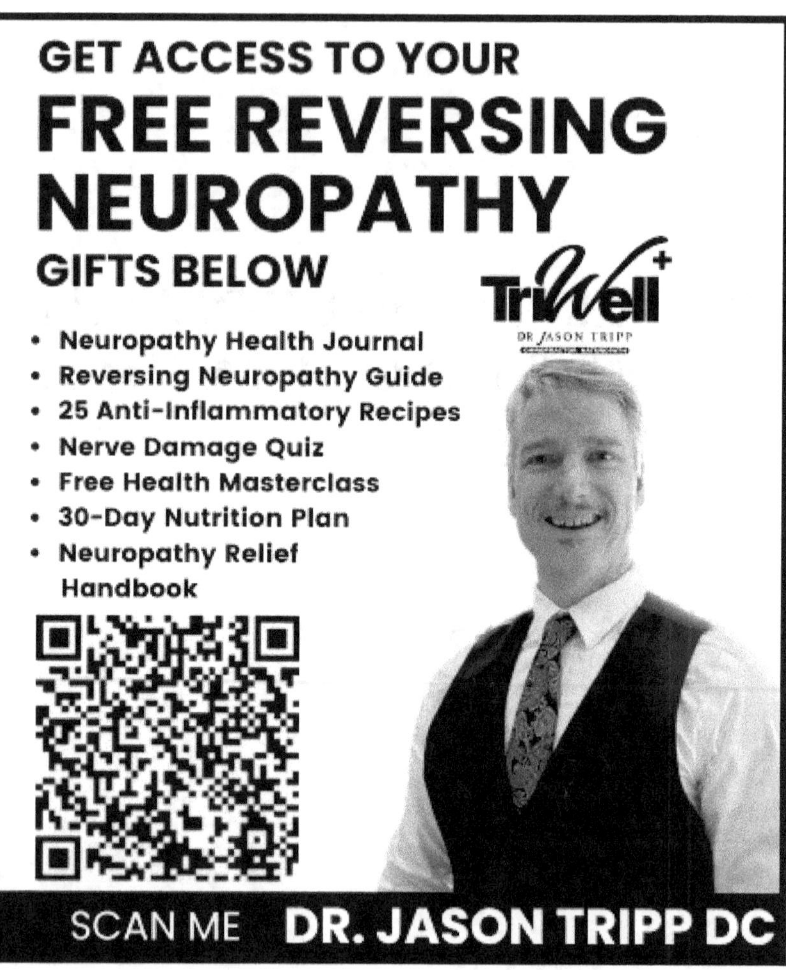

Unlock your Path to Relief Now: Dial (724) 342-2225 to speak with a Neuropathy Care Specialist Today!

CONTENTS

FOREWORD

Neuropathy is often considered a life sentence – an ongoing struggle with pain, numbness, and discomfort that slowly chips away at one's quality of life. Yet, as countless patients have discovered through the dedication and expertise of Dr. Jason Tripp, this doesn't have to be the case.

Dr. Tripp, a fellow chiropractic practitioner, a colleague within the Driven Doc community at The Data Driven Practice, and a true pioneer in the field of neuropathy treatment, has consistently demonstrated that reversal is possible. His innovative TriWell Nerve F.R.E.E.D.O.M. Program, the cornerstone of this groundbreaking book, is a testament to his unwavering commitment to patient care and his relentless pursuit of effective, holistic solutions.

Within these pages, Dr. Tripp shares the culmination of his extensive research, clinical experience, and unwavering passion for helping those suffering from neuropathy. "Reversing Neuropathy: The F.R.E.E.D.O.M. Method" is not simply a guidebook; it's a beacon of hope, a roadmap to reclaiming control of one's health, and a testament to the power of integrative medicine.

I've had the privilege of witnessing firsthand the transformative impact of Dr. Tripp's FREEDOM Method. The results speak for themselves, as patients once resigned to a life of chronic pain rediscover the joy of movement, sensation, and overall well-being. This book is a gift to anyone seeking a way out of the darkness of neuropathy, offering a clear path towards freedom from pain and a life lived to the fullest.

Dr. Tripp and his exceptional team at Tripp Chiropractic & Nutrition are more than just healthcare providers; they are partners in your journey toward healing. This book is your first step. Embrace the knowledge within, follow the guidance provided, and reclaim the vibrant, pain-free life you deserve.

Dr. Cory Frogley

The Data Driven Practice

ABOUT THE AUTHOR

I'm Dr. Jason Tripp, and my story begins not in a lab coat, but in a church pew. At five years old, I felt a deep calling to help people heal naturally, guided by God's hand. This wasn't just a childhood dream; it became a life-defining mission, fueled by a personal journey of pain and triumph.

At 17, a horrific car accident shattered my spine, leaving me with seven herniated discs and a twenty-five-year battle with chronic pain. The agony seeped beyond my back, manifesting as headaches, digestive woes, fatigue, and eventually, a debilitating case of neuropathy. My feet, once instruments of movement, became searing embers. Each step felt like walking on fire.

But even in the darkest hours, the call to heal remained. I devoured knowledge, accumulating eight degrees, 125 certificates, and a relentless thirst for understanding. One fateful training program presented a beacon of hope: the secrets to reversing neuropathy. With meticulous dedication, I applied these principles, not just to neuropathy, but to the constellation of ailments plaguing me.

And then, the miracle arrived. My pain subsided, replaced by a newfound vibrancy. This wasn't a fluke, but a testament to the transformative power of holistic healing. I couldn't keep this knowledge to myself. It was time to share the F.R.E.E.D.O.M. method, a holistic system born from my own struggles, refined through years of research, and imbued with the unwavering belief that healing is possible.

This isn't just a book about neuropathy; it's a roadmap to reclaiming your health, and your life. I hope this book will inspire and help those who are suffering from chronic health conditions. Thank you for joining me on this journey.

THE NEUROPATHY CRISIS

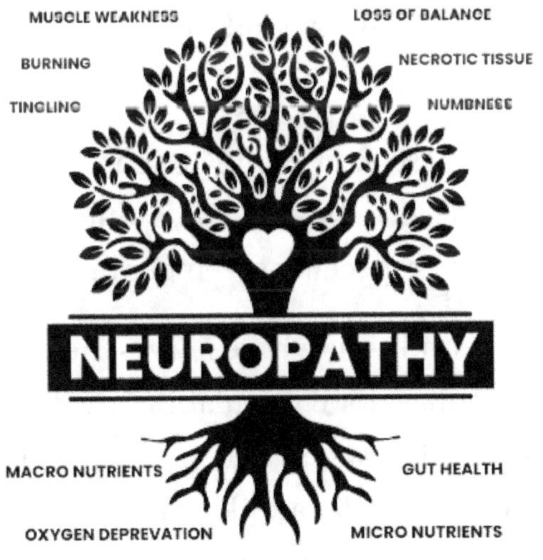

Amazing Transformation: Rose

In January, Rose came to see me concerning her neuropathy symptoms. She was extremely worried about the condition of her legs and feet. Rose experienced severe pain, itching, numbness, and tingling. Walking was challenging due to her lack of balance, and she felt herself deteriorating rapidly.

The symptoms seemed to appear out of nowhere. The pain was so excruciating that she had to walk on the sides of her feet because putting weight on the soles was unbearable. Her feet felt as hard as rocks. She observed a severe lack of blood circulation in her legs and feet, which appeared pale and devoid of the normal reddish hue.

Rose feared the worst, expressing her concern that she might have to undergo a bilateral foot amputation, a terrifying prospect, especially given her diabetic condition.

Neuropathy is a condition where nerves die off due to a loss of microvascular blood circulation. Healthy nerves require ample blood flow, and when this is compromised, the nerve begins to deteriorate. This is when symptoms like pain, numbness, itching, burning, cramping, temperature sensitivity, and unusual sensations like bunched-up socks or crawling bugs manifest.

Neuropathy is a progressive and degenerative condition, meaning it worsens over time if left untreated. It can progress from mild to severe or even permanent, and in many cases, it can lead to amputation.

I developed the TriWell Nerve F.R.E.E.D.O.M. Program, a holistic approach that treats the individual as a whole. This system recognizes that we are mental, emotional, and spiritual beings with physical bodies that require proper nourishment. Neuropathy has over a hundred different potential causes, which can be categorized into three groups: neurological (brain, spinal nerves, and peripheral nerves), structural (ligaments, muscles, and tendons), and metabolic (gut health, nutritional deficiencies, and toxicity). In the FREEDOM Program, we test for all three categories of neuropathy causes – neurological, structural, and metabolic.

When you identify the exact cause of your problem, finding a solution becomes much easier. When you know precisely what you need to do based on scientific testing tailored to your specific needs, it becomes easier to commit to doing whatever it takes to recover.

Rose understood this and became committed to following the program diligently. She did exactly as instructed, and by the end of January, she had already started seeing improvements.

Within 3-4 weeks, the changes were noticeable. The tingling and numbness had almost disappeared, and her feet had regained their soft, normal texture.

Encouraged by the positive results, she remained dedicated to the recommended therapy.

Rose had previously experienced tingling throughout her entire right side, but by this time, the numbness and tingling in her right arm had completely subsided. She was amazed at the rapidity of her progress.

By March, Rose exclaimed about her results, "It's amazing—unbelievable that everything is getting better! I used to be on a C-PAP machine for 6 years. I've been off it for 3 months now, going on 4 months. I used to stop breathing in my sleep. Now, I can breathe without it!

I'm amazed at my feet. They're awesome! They're red, and blood is flowing! They're not all white and hard like rocks anymore. It's amazing how this therapy has really helped me. It's working! You stick to all the therapy Dr. Tripp recommends because you know you're getting better and better. I love it. I'm so excited! People ask me about it all the time – they want the number whenever I tell my story. I get asked every day and pass along Dr. Tripp's number to their uncle, mother, or themselves... I share it with anyone who asks."

Understanding Peripheral Neuropathy

Imagine waking up to a relentless tingling in your feet, a sensation that persists throughout the day and makes even the simplest tasks feel like impossible challenges.

This is just one of the many faces of peripheral neuropathy, a condition that affects the peripheral nerves, the intricate network that connects our central nervous system to the rest of our body. They carry messages that control the sensations, movements, and functions of your organs and systems.

Peripheral neuropathy can affect three types of peripheral nerves:

- **Sensory nerves**, which carry information about touch, pain, temperature, or pressure from your skin and other tissues to your brain
- **Motor nerves**, which carry information from your brain to your muscles and control your voluntary movements, such as walking, typing, or lifting
- **Autonomic nerves**, which carry information from your brain to your organs and glands and control your involuntary functions, such as digestion, urination, sexual function, or blood pressure

Depending on which type of peripheral nerve is damaged and how severely, you may experience different symptoms of peripheral neuropathy. For example, if your sensory nerves are affected, you may feel pain, burning, tingling, or numbness in your hands, feet, or other parts of your body. If your motor nerves are affected, you may have muscle weakness, cramps, spasms, or twitching. And if your autonomic nerves are affected, you may have problems with digestion, urination, sexual function, or blood pressure.

To illustrate what someone with peripheral neuropathy might go through in their daily life, let me share with you the story of a patient named John. John is a 45-year-old accountant who was diagnosed with type 2 diabetes ten years ago. He has been managing his blood sugar levels with medication and diet, but he hasn't been very consistent or careful.

About a year ago, he started to notice some strange sensations in his feet. He felt like he was walking on pins and needles or wearing socks that were too tight. He also felt some sharp pains that would come and go or some coldness that would not go away. He ignored these symptoms, thinking they were just minor annoyances or signs of aging.

But over time, his symptoms got worse. He started to lose feeling in his feet, and he could not tell if he was stepping on something sharp or if his shoes were too loose. He also developed some sores and blisters on his feet that he didn't notice until they became infected.

He also had trouble walking, as his feet felt heavy and clumsy. He stumbled and fell several times and injured himself. He also had difficulty sleeping, as his feet would keep him awake at night. He became depressed and anxious and lost interest in his work and hobbies.

He finally decided to see a doctor, who diagnosed him with diabetic peripheral neuropathy, a type of peripheral neuropathy that affects about 50% of people with diabetes. His doctor explained that his high blood sugar levels had damaged his peripheral nerves, especially the sensory and motor nerves in his feet.

His doctor prescribed him some painkillers and antidepressants and advised him to take better care of his diabetes and his feet and said there was not much else that they could do.

John was shocked and scared by his diagnosis, and he felt hopeless and helpless. He wondered if he would ever get better or if he would lose his feet or his legs. He wondered if he would ever be able to enjoy his life again or if he would be a burden to his family and friends. He felt alone and isolated and did not know where to turn for help.

John's story is not uncommon. Many people with peripheral neuropathy go through similar experiences and face similar challenges. Peripheral neuropathy is not only a physical condition but also a psychological and social one. It can significantly impact your health and well-being and affect your personal, professional, and social life.

According to the World Health Organization, peripheral neuropathy affects about 8% of the global population and is one of the leading causes of disability. Peripheral neuropathy can also increase your risk of developing other complications, such as infections, ulcers, amputations, falls, fractures, depression, anxiety, or suicide.

But there is hope. Peripheral neuropathy is not a life sentence. You can reverse it, or at least improve it, by following the FREEDOM method, a holistic, non-invasive three-step program I've developed and refined over the years based on my extensive research and clinical experience.

The FREEDOM method will help you heal your nerves and reclaim your life by finding and addressing the root cause of your neuropathy, eliminating inflammation, soothing pain, teaching your nerves to communicate effectively once more, oxygenating your tissues, restoring your mobility and balance, and elevating your quality of life.

But before we dive into the FREEDOM program, there are some important actions that you need to take to understand your peripheral neuropathy better and prepare yourself for the healing journey. These actions are:

- **Identify your symptoms early.** The earlier you detect your symptoms of peripheral neuropathy, the better your chances of reversing or improving it. Don't ignore or dismiss your symptoms, as they may indicate nerve damage that can worsen over time. Pay attention to any changes in your sensations, movements, or functions, and report them to your doctor as soon as possible.

- **Document your symptom patterns**. Keeping a record of your symptoms can help you and your doctor understand your peripheral neuropathy better and find the best treatment plan for you. You can use a journal, a calendar, or an app to track your symptoms, such as when they occur, how long they last, how severe they are, what triggers or relieves them, and how they affect your daily activities and quality of life.

You can also note any other factors that may be related to your peripheral neuropathy, such as your blood sugar levels, medications, diet, exercise, stress, or sleep.

- **Seek regular medical check-ups**. Seeing a holistic doctor regularly can help you monitor your peripheral neuropathy and prevent or treat any complications that may arise. We can perform various tests to assess your nerve function. We can also prescribe non-addictive supplements or complementary therapies to help you manage your symptoms.
- **Stay informed**. Educating yourself about peripheral neuropathy can help you better

understand your condition and empower you to take charge of your health. You can learn more about peripheral neuropathy from other books, websites, podcasts, or videos. You can also join support groups, online forums, or social media platforms to connect with other people with peripheral neuropathy and share your experiences, insights, or tips. You can also ask questions, seek advice, or get feedback from a neuropathy specialist who can provide professional guidance and support.

The Progression of Neuropathy

One of the things that you need to understand about peripheral neuropathy is that it is not a static condition. It is a dynamic and progressive condition that can change over time and affect different body parts and aspects of your life.

In this section, I'll explain what the progression of neuropathy means and how it can vary greatly among individuals. I'll also share with you some examples of how the progression of neuropathy can affect your daily life and what you can do to prevent or slow down its progression and preserve your quality of life and independence.

The progression of neuropathy refers to how your symptoms of nerve damage change over time in terms of their intensity, frequency, duration, or spread. Initially, your symptoms may be mild, like occasional tingling or numbness in your fingers or toes. You may not even notice them or think they're typical signs of aging or caused by something else, like cold weather, tight shoes, or poor posture. So, you may not feel the need to seek medical attention or to do anything about them.

But over time, your symptoms may get worse. They may become more intense, more frequent, more persistent, or more widespread. You may start to feel pain, burning, or electric shocks in your hands, feet, or other parts of your body. You may lose feeling in your affected areas and have trouble sensing touch, temperature, or pressure. You may also have problems with your muscle strength, balance, coordination, or reflexes.

You may have difficulty walking, driving, working, or taking care of yourself or others. You may also develop other complications, such as infections, ulcers, amputations, falls, fractures, or depression.

Consider Michael's story. It began with a mild tingling in his toes, a sensation that gradually crept upwards, transforming into agonizing burning sensations. This progression significantly impacted his mobility, making even simple walks a challenge. Similarly, another patient, Emma, started with occasional tingling in her hands, gradually progressing to a noticeable decline in her ability to grasp objects firmly.

The progression of neuropathy can have profound consequences, including chronic pain, impaired mobility, and increased risk of injury. Recognizing and addressing symptoms early is crucial to slow or even halt their progression, preserving quality of life and independence.

Here are some action steps that you can take to manage the progression of your neuropathy:

- **Monitor your symptoms regularly**. Be vigilant about any changes in your symptoms' intensity, frequency, duration, or spread. Don't ignore or dismiss your symptoms, as they may indicate nerve damage that can worsen over time. Pay attention to any changes in your sensations, movements, or functions, and report them to your doctor as soon as possible.
- **Maintain regular communication with your healthcare providers**. Schedule regular check-ups with your healthcare provider to discuss any changes you've noticed and receive ongoing guidance on managing your condition.
- **Adapt lifestyle changes**. Making some adjustments to your diet, exercise, stress, or sleep can be beneficial for your nerve health and your overall health. For example, eating a balanced and nutritious diet rich in antioxidants, anti-inflammatory, and nerve-protective foods can help

lower your blood sugar, reduce inflammation, and support and repair your nerve function.

Exercising regularly, with low-impact and moderate-intensity activities like walking, swimming, or cycling, can help you improve your blood circulation, oxygen delivery, muscle strength, balance, and mood. Managing your stress with relaxation techniques, such as meditation, yoga, or breathing exercises, can help you lower your cortisol levels, which can damage your nerves.

Getting enough sleep, with good sleep hygiene, such as avoiding caffeine, alcohol, or screens before bed, can help restore your energy, repair your nerves, and regulate your hormones.

- **Stay proactive in your treatment**. Don't rely solely on traditional treatments, such as addictive medications that may only mask your symptoms. Explore other holistic, natural options, such as supplements or acupuncture, that can offer you natural and effective solutions for your peripheral neuropathy.

Supplements, such as alpha-lipoic acid, acetyl-L-carnitine, or B vitamins, can help you improve your nerve function, reduce your nerve pain, and protect your nerves from further damage. Acupuncture can help you stimulate your nerve endings, increase your blood flow, release your endorphins, and balance your energy.

The Limitations of Traditional Approaches

For many individuals battling peripheral neuropathy, the journey toward relief often involves a whirlwind of traditional treatment options, each offering a glimmer of hope yet falling short of a lasting solution.

While medications may provide temporary pain relief, they often come with a slew of side effects and do little to address the underlying causes of neuropathy. Similarly, physical therapy and surgery, while sometimes beneficial, can offer only temporary respite from symptoms, leaving individuals feeling trapped in a cycle of recurring pain and discomfort.

Just take a look at Linda's experience, a neuropathic patient who was initially prescribed pain medication for her neuropathic pain, but the relief was only temporary. The medication soon became less effective, and the side effects grew more pronounced, leaving her feeling more burdened than before.

It's the same story with Mike, another neuropathy patient. After undergoing surgery, he found the relief fleeting, with symptoms resurfacing and leaving him questioning the long-term efficacy of this approach.

These experiences highlight the limitations of relying solely on traditional neuropathy treatments. The focus on symptom management, while offering temporary relief, fails to address the root causes of the condition, leading to a cycle of recurring symptoms and potential dependency on medications. This approach can significantly diminish overall quality of life and hinder individuals' ability to live fulfilling lives.

The limitations of traditional neuropathy treatments underscore the need for a more comprehensive and holistic approach. In simpler terms, a holistic approach means treating the whole you, not just the symptoms. It considers how different aspects of your life – your diet, stress levels, sleep patterns – can all work together to influence your neuropathy and your overall health.

By going deeper into the underlying causes of neuropathy, we can unlock more sustainable and effective solutions that address the root of the problem, not just its symptoms.

It's time to move beyond accepting temporary fixes as the only solution. Question the effectiveness of treatments that provide fleeting relief without addressing the root of the condition. Seek alternatives that offer long-term benefits and restore your overall health and well-being.

If your current neuropathy treatment plan isn't giving you the desired results you're looking for, don't hesitate to seek second opinions. Consult with different healthcare providers to explore a wider range of treatment options and gain a broader perspective on your condition.

Try to learn more about holistic treatments that focus on overall health and root causes. These approaches include dietary modifications, acupuncture, chiropractic care, and stress management techniques, all aimed at promoting overall well-being and creating an environment conducive to healing, which is really what the TriWell Nerve FREEDOM Program is all about. By addressing the root causes of neuropathy, FREEDOM offers a more sustainable and effective path to long-term relief and improved quality of life.

Remember, the journey towards effective neuropathy treatment is not a one-size-fits-all approach. By questioning the status quo, seeking second opinions, and exploring holistic approaches, you can empower yourself to find the most suitable path toward sustainable relief and enhanced well-being.

When Neuropathy Becomes Critical

When peripheral neuropathy escalates beyond manageable discomfort and significantly disrupts daily life, things get critical. It's often marked by intense, unrelenting pain that defies conventional pain management strategies. The loss of sensation in the hands or feet can lead to frequent falls and injuries, while mobility issues can hinder independence and drastically alter one's lifestyle.

Imagine reaching the point where you can no longer feel your feet, leading to a cascade of falls and injuries. Or picture neuropathy-related pain so severe that it disrupts sleep, worsens anxiety, and diminishes your overall mental health. These scenarios highlight the profound implications of neuropathy reaching a critical stage.

The consequences of critical neuropathy extend far beyond physical discomfort. The increased risk of injuries due to diminished sensation can lead to a reliance on others for assistance, potentially robbing individuals of their independence. Moreover, the relentless pain and challenges posed by neuropathy can significantly impact one's mental health, leading to anxiety, depression, and social isolation.

Therefore, addressing neuropathy before it reaches a critical stage is crucial for maintaining independence, quality of life, and overall well-being. Regular health assessments, including neurological examinations, can help identify early signs of worsening symptoms, allowing for timely intervention.

If you experience a sudden intensification of symptoms, such as increased pain, loss of sensation, or mobility issues, seek medical attention. Don't wait for it to become critical. Early intervention can prevent further nerve damage and potentially reverse the progression of neuropathy.

Adopting healthy lifestyle choices, such as a balanced diet, regular exercise, and stress management techniques, can reduce the risk factors associated with neuropathy. These measures promote overall health and create an environment conducive to nerve function.

Navigating the challenges of neuropathy can take a toll on one's mental health. Seeking counseling or therapy can provide emotional support, coping strategies, and tools for managing stress and anxiety, empowering individuals to thrive despite their condition.

Early intervention and a holistic approach to treatment are vital to preventing neuropathy from reaching a critical stage. By staying vigilant, responding promptly to changes, adopting preventive measures, and seeking mental health support, you can empower yourself to reclaim your quality of life and navigate the journey of neuropathy with resilience and hope.

ACTION STEP: Start a daily journal of your symptoms. This will allow you to more accurately sense your level of improvement when starting a neuropathy treatment regimen.

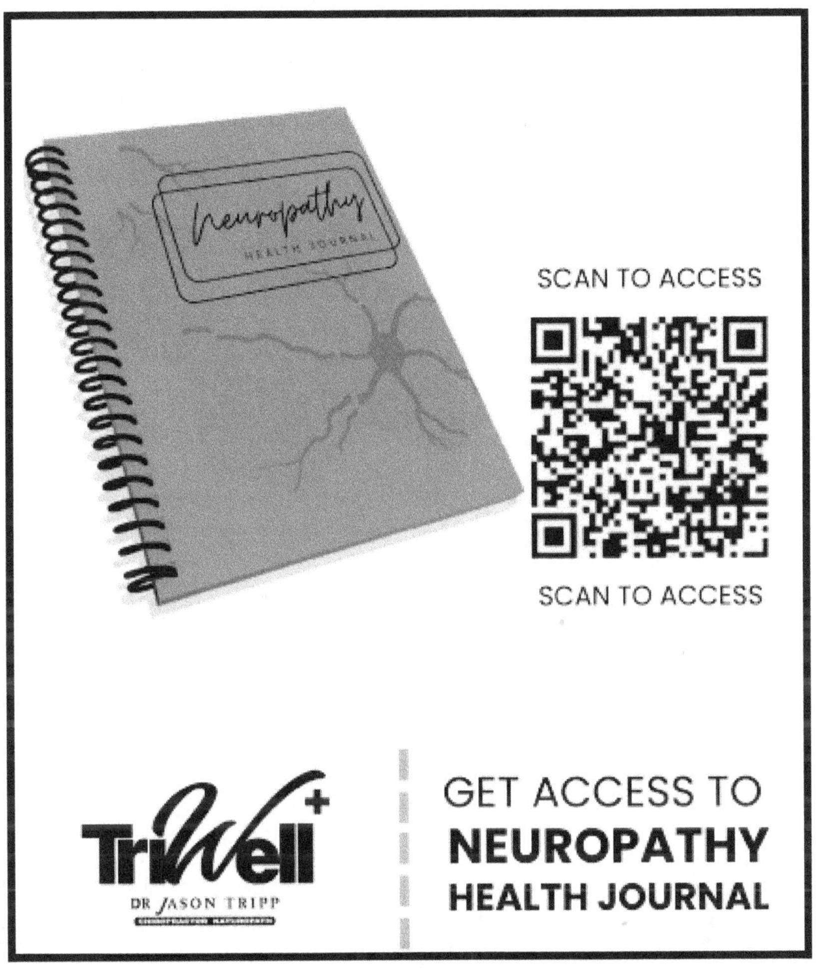

Unlock your Path to Relief Now: Dial (724) 342-2225 to speak with a Neuropathy Care Specialist Today!

2

———

THE PROMISE OF F.R.E.E.D.O.M

Jeanie's Incredible Neuropathy Healing Journey

Jeanie came to my office with severe neuropathy symptoms. Initially, I wasn't sure if I could help her. As part of our Neuropathy FREEDOM examination, we determine whether we can assist a patient based on our exam findings. This exam includes a neuropathy severity test to assess the extent of the neuropathy and determine if we can provide effective treatment. If the patient has more than 85% damage to the peripheral nerves in the hands or feet, we may be unable to help. However, if the patient has 85% damage or less, we can likely provide relief. Fortunately, Jeanie's condition fell within the treatable range. She has an amazing testimony about her experience with the NEUROPATHY FREEDOM program, which I'll let her share in her own words.

"My name is Jeanie. I've been having problems with my feet for 20 years. Four doctors turned me down and wouldn't even discuss what was happening. I saw the advertisement on TV after returning from a vacation with my family. My son told me that everyone was looking at me like I was drunk or full of beer. I explained that it had to do with my feet. That's when I decided to see Dr. Tripp. I came here, and I was a little hesitant. I didn't know if I could be helped or not. I told him I was so damaged that I didn't think I could be repaired. He assured me, 'Yes, you can – you can be repaired.'

"So far, I've been here for 5 weeks. Last Sunday was the first time I could walk up the aisle at my church to receive communion. I'm so proud of myself! I'm also getting good sleep. My feet aren't cold anymore. I don't have to use 4 blankets and 2 pairs of socks. I can sleep like a baby for eight hours straight with just one blanket. I would highly recommend Dr. Tripp. The people who work here take care of me. They are wonderful. They treat you like an individual, not a number. They treat you like their mother, grandmother, or sister. They are really wonderful people. If you have a problem with your feet and your doctors are dismissing you, take advantage of the offer on TV. Take it to heart. It's just a phone call. You won't regret it."

A New Dawn for Neuropathy Patients

The TriWell Nerve FREEDOM Program is like a skilled gardener tending to a neglected orchard. Instead of simply picking up fallen fruit (treating symptoms), this program nurtures the roots and branches of your nervous system. It recognizes that neuropathy isn't just an isolated event, but a sign of deeper imbalances. By restoring the vitality of your nerves, this program isn't just offering a band-aid; it's cultivating a thriving ecosystem of well-being where neuropathy struggles to take root.

How Dr. Tripp Saved My Feet and My Life: Dave's Story

For many years, I dealt with the pain and numbness of neuropathy in both of my feet. All my previous doctor could do was offer medication to "manage" the pain, but nothing to correct the problem. Eventually I would have lost the ability to walk.

Dr. Tripp offered his FREEDOM program to repair the damaged nerves. I've only been on the program for three months, but I have experienced remarkable progress. I no longer have pain in my feet, and the sensation of touch is slowly returning.

I also suffered from a continuous headache for nearly three years due to damage to my neck. After a CAT scan, I was told it was just from age and to put warm compresses on it to soothe it. Again, no offer to correct the problem. In just one session in which my neck was "cracked" by Dr. Tripp, my headache disappeared. It still returns from time to time, but with less severity and only for a few hours.

I managed my pain for many years, adding more and more medications to a daily regimen just to "take the edge off." Dr. Tripp has shown me a better alternative.

Transformative Healing: Reclaiming Your Life from Neuropathy

Transformative healing in the context of neuropathy is not just about easing symptoms or managing the condition; it's about setting out on a journey of profound and lasting change in your health and well-being.

The FREEDOM method empowers you to achieve this transformation by addressing the multifaceted nature of neuropathy, encompassing physical symptoms, underlying health issues, and lifestyle factors.

Imagine a life where neuropathy doesn't dictate your every move, where the pain that once held you back is now a distant memory, where you can walk, run, and engage in activities you once loved without fear of falling or enduring discomfort. This is the promise of transformative healing with the FREEDOM method.

While transformative healing requires dedication and consistent effort, the rewards far outweigh the investment. Patients who fully embrace the FREEDOM method often experience:

- **Reduced pain and improved mobility**: The method addresses the underlying causes of neuropathy, leading to a significant decrease in pain and an enhanced ability to move freely.

- **Enhanced mental health**: The holistic approach of the FREEDOM method promotes overall well-being, alleviating anxiety, depression, and fatigue associated with neuropathy.
- **A renewed sense of hope**: As symptoms improve and overall well-being is enhanced, individuals regain a sense of control over their lives and a renewed optimism for the future.

The cost of not pursuing transformative healing is a continuation of suffering, a diminished quality of life, and the possibility of irreversible nerve damage.

By choosing the comprehensive approach of the FREEDOM method, you invest in your long-term health and well-being, empowering yourself to reclaim the life you deserve.

Embracing a Holistic Approach

Transformative healing is a journey, not a destination. It requires a commitment to comprehensive change, encompassing physical, mental, and emotional aspects of your well-being. Here are some steps you can take to embrace holistic healing:

- **Commit to the FREEDOM method in its entirety**: Follow the program's guidelines, attend all sessions, and actively participate in the recommended activities.

- **Monitor your symptoms and overall well-being**: Keep a journal to track your progress, noting any improvements or changes in symptoms.
- **Incorporate healthy dietary and exercise habits**: Nourish your body with nutrient-rich foods and engage in regular physical activity to promote overall health and support nerve regeneration.
- **Seek support when needed**: Use support groups or therapy to address any mental or emotional challenges that may arise during your healing journey.

Remember, transformative healing is a collaborative effort. Work closely with the Tripp Chiropractic & Nutrition team, ask questions, and express any concerns you may have along the way. Together, we can navigate the path of profound healing, reclaiming your health, vitality, and fulfilling life that is rightfully yours.

Beyond Symptom Management

When it comes to neuropathy, the common approach often centers on symptom management, aiming to provide temporary relief from pain and discomfort. While this may offer some immediate respite, it fails to address the underlying causes of neuropathy, leaving individuals trapped in a cycle of recurring symptoms and potential dependency on medications.

The FREEDOM method breaks free from this reactive pattern, moving beyond symptom management to embrace a holistic approach that tackles the root causes of neuropathy and promotes long-term healing and restoration.

This comprehensive strategy recognizes that neuropathy is not just a symptom but a complex condition influenced by a multitude of factors, including genetics, lifestyle choices, and underlying health conditions. Armed with this comprehensive understanding of neuropathy's far-reaching causes, the journey toward sustainable healing can commence.

It begins with understanding the unique factors contributing to your neuropathy. This may involve exploring your medical history, assessing lifestyle habits, and undergoing diagnostic tests to identify any underlying health conditions.

By gaining a deeper understanding of the root causes, we can tailor your treatment plan to address these specific issues and prevent further nerve damage.

Developing a holistic treatment plan requires a collaborative effort that should encompass a range of therapeutic modalities, including:

- **Dietary modifications**: Nourish your body with nutrient-rich foods that support nerve health and promote overall well-being.

- **Stress management techniques**: Implement practices like mindfulness, yoga, or meditation to reduce stress, a significant contributor to neuropathy.
- **Physical therapy**: Engage in targeted exercises and physical therapy to improve muscle strength, balance, and mobility.
- **Complementary therapies**: Explore acupuncture, chiropractic care, or other complementary therapies that may provide additional benefits.

Lifestyle changes also play a pivotal role in supporting healing and promoting long-term health. Consider adopting healthier habits such as:

- **Regular exercise**: Engage in moderate-intensity physical activity most days of the week to promote nerve health and overall well-being.
- **Balanced diet**: Consume a nutrient-rich diet rich in fruits, vegetables, whole grains, and lean protein sources.
- **Adequate sleep**: Prioritize quality sleep to allow your body to rest, repair, and rejuvenate.
- **Smoking cessation**: Quitting smoking can significantly reduce the risk of neuropathy progression and improve overall health.

Keep a journal to track your symptoms, lifestyle changes, and any improvements or challenges you encounter. Communicate openly with your healthcare providers, discuss any concerns, and seek guidance in refining your treatment approach.

By moving beyond symptom management and embracing a holistic approach, you empower yourself to address the underlying causes of neuropathy, promote long-term healing, and reclaim your quality of life.

While holistic therapies and supplements are crucial in managing neuropathy, the wellness journey extends far beyond the doctor's office. It's about taking control of your health and well-being and making conscious choices that support your overall well-being, which includes adopting healthy dietary habits, incorporating regular exercise into your routine, and implementing stress management techniques like mindfulness or meditation.

Combined with other treatments, these lifestyle changes can significantly improve your neuropathy symptoms, boost your energy levels, and enhance your overall quality of life.

The Power of Support and Guidance

The journey to wellness is not a solo endeavor. It's about surrounding yourself with a supportive network that encourages and uplifts you along the way. Joining support groups can connect you with others who understand your challenges and provide invaluable peer-to-peer support.

Healthcare professionals, such as chiropractors, acupuncturists, and physical therapists, can provide personalized guidance and expertise to help you achieve your health goals. Wellness coaches can offer additional support, helping you stay motivated, overcome obstacles, and celebrate your progress.

The path to wellness is a journey, not a destination. It's about making consistent efforts, embracing healthy habits, and celebrating achievements, no matter how small. Acknowledge the progress you've made, no matter how incremental. Each step forward is a step towards a healthier, happier you.

Debbie's Triumph: Overcoming Numbness and Embracing Sensation

"I've been coming to Dr. Tripp for three weeks, and when I first came, I had a lot of numbness in my hands. I didn't realize until today how long it had been since I felt my fingers. It was actually right after the first session, and I just want to tell Dr. Tripp, thank you very much."

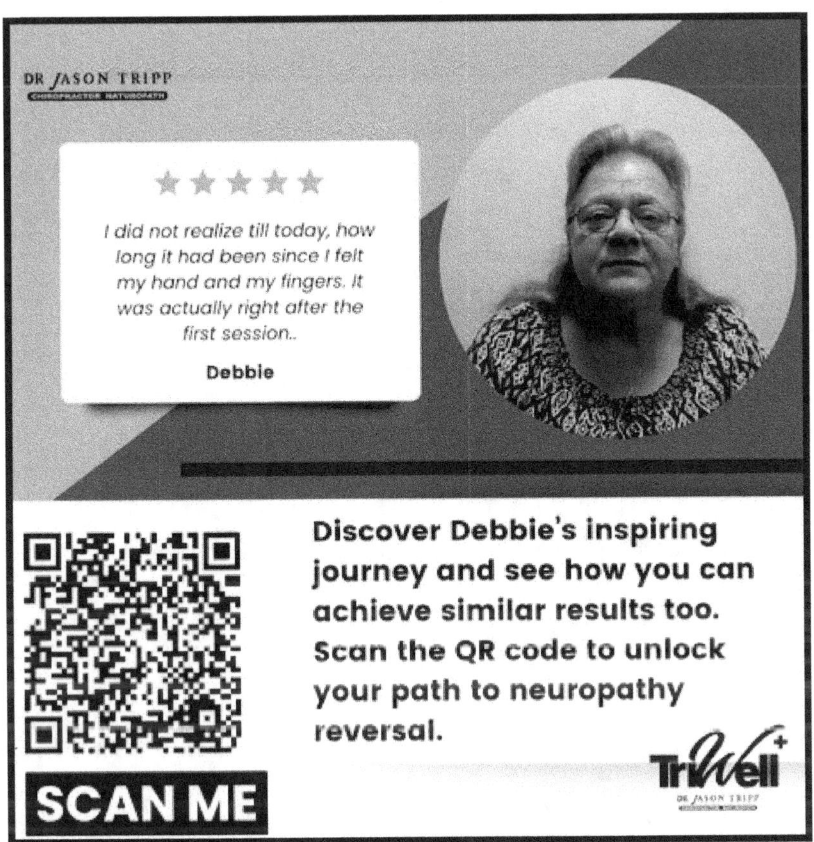

Unlock your Path to Relief Now: Dial (724) 342-2225 to speak with a Neuropathy Care Specialist Today!

3

DEBUNKING NEUROPATHY MYTHS

Many people are mistakenly told that neuropathy is an irreversible condition. Sylvia's story serves as a prime example of how this myth is false. Sylvia came to Tripp Chiropractic seeking relief from her debilitating neuropathy symptoms. She suffered from neuropathy in both hands and feet. Her doctor had prescribed an EMG test, which confirmed she had severe neuropathy. Sylvia described the sensation in her feet as feeling like she was walking on rocks or marbles, making it exhausting to move around. The neuropathy pain was a staggering 9 out of 10. She was in constant, excruciating pain, which had been ongoing for over 18 years in her feet and over 28 years in her hands.

The condition began to affect all aspects of her health and life. She struggled with walking and sleeping. Her ability to go places was limited by how she felt on any given day. Sylvia lamented, "I had lost all enjoyment in going places and doing things. It just hurt too much." Basic tasks like grocery shopping or running errands became increasingly difficult. When she pushed through the pain to go somewhere or do something, she would be left in agony for days afterward. Lying down at night to sleep only exacerbated her discomfort, making it extremely challenging to get restful sleep.

Sylvia tried various remedies to alleviate the pain, including Pilates, which she eventually had to stop because the pain became too severe even to put on her shoes. She exhausted all options: Neurontin, Gabapentin, Lyrica, Cymbalta, Physical Therapy, pain medications, over-the-counter remedies, injections, creams – you name it, she tried it. But nothing provided relief, and she continued to suffer. "It was year after year of SUFFERING!" she exclaimed. "It made me not want to even try. I was losing my freedom. And I was not okay with that... but didn't know what to do to change it." The loss of sleep, enjoyment of life, and freedom was taking a severe toll. After years of lost time and quality of life, she had almost given up on finding help since nothing she tried provided answers or relief. She needed help desperately.

That's when Sylvia came to my office, and upon examination, she had one of the most severe cases of neuropathy. As part of our Neuropathy FREEDOM examination, we conduct a neuropathy severity test to determine the extent of the condition and whether we can provide effective treatment. If the patient has more than 85% damage to the peripheral nerves in the hands or feet, we may be unable to help. However, if the patient has 85% damage or less, we can likely provide relief. When I tested Sylvia, she was at 85% – right at the edge of being unable to be helped.

We started care immediately since time was against Sylvia. If her condition worsened, it could become irreversible. I recommended a comprehensive neuropathy program to help her feel better, regain her life, and reclaim her FREEDOM. She diligently followed everything I instructed, and the results have been amazing. Sylvia reported that her neuropathy symptoms improved significantly. Week by week, she kept getting better and better. She exclaimed that her neuropathy was no longer at the brink of being untreatable, and she felt remarkably better. Sylvia declared, "I'm so glad I was led to Tripp Chiropractic & Nutrition. I'm happy with Dr. Tripp and the entire staff." What an incredible transformation! She went from losing all quality of life to pain, suffering, and being unable to live the way she wanted – in freedom. Now, she has FREEDOM from neuropathy and FREEDOM to get back to living the life of her dreams.

Now the world of neuropathy treatment is often clouded with misconceptions and myths that can hinder effective care and prevent individuals from seeking the relief they deserve. So this chapter aims to shed light on the realities of neuropathy, separating fact from fiction and empowering you to make informed decisions about your health.

Myth: Neuropathy is always irreversible.

This is a prevalent misconception that can instill a sense of hopelessness and resignation among neuropathy patients. However, the truth is that neuropathy can indeed be reversed or significantly improved, especially when addressed early and with a comprehensive approach.

Our patient, Andres, exemplifies this. Despite facing severe neuropathy and a significant loss of sensation in his feet, he regained his mobility and became pain-free through the FREEDOM method.

After his first treatment, he said that he felt his toes for the first time in "I don't know how long." His story serves as a beacon of hope, demonstrating that neuropathy doesn't have to dictate one's future.

Myth: Neuropathy only affects the elderly.

While neuropathy is more common in older individuals, it's not limited to that age group. Younger individuals can also develop neuropathy due to various factors, including genetic predisposition, autoimmune disorders, and certain medications. It's crucial to dispel this myth and recognize that neuropathy can affect anyone at any age.

Myth: Neuropathy is just a symptom of diabetes.

Neuropathy is a complex condition with multiple potential causes, not just diabetes. While diabetes is a significant risk factor for neuropathy, it's not the sole cause. Other underlying conditions, such as vitamin deficiencies, autoimmune diseases, and nerve compression, can also contribute to neuropathy.

Myth: Neuropathy only presents as pain.

Neuropathy can manifest in various ways, including numbness, tingling, weakness, burning sensation, and balance problems. Pain is a common symptom, but it's not the only one.

Myth: I just have to live with neuropathy.

You don't have to accept neuropathy as an inevitable part of your life. With proper treatment, lifestyle modifications, and a proactive approach to your health, you can take control of your neuropathy, manage your symptoms effectively, and reclaim your quality of life.

Believing in these myths can have very harmful

consequences for neuropathy patients. It can lead to despair, discouragement, and a delay in seeking effective care. They also fall victim to ineffective treatments or therapies that promise miraculous cures but fail to address the underlying causes of their neuropathy.

Understanding the realities of neuropathy is the first step towards effective treatment and improved quality of life. Here are some actions you can take to empower yourself with knowledge:

- **Challenge common misconceptions**: Discuss your concerns or doubts about neuropathy with a specialist. They can help you separate fact from fiction and provide accurate information.
- **Educate yourself**: Stay up-to-date on the latest research and advancements in neuropathy treatment. Read credible sources, attend patient education workshops like the ones we regularly have at drjasontripp.com, and engage in online forums to gather reliable information. Here are links to a few credible sources:
- Mayo Clinic
- MedlinePlus
- Department of Health and Human Services (HHS)
- Centers for Disease Control and Prevention (CDC)
- American Medical Association (AMA)
- National Institutes of Health (NIH)

- **Share accurate information**: Help others by spreading awareness about the realities of neuropathy. Educate your family, friends, and community about the condition, dispel myths, and encourage them to seek appropriate care.
- **Stay open to new treatments**: Be receptive to emerging therapies and approaches in neuropathy treatment. While exercising caution and making informed decisions is important, don't let fear or skepticism prevent you from exploring potentially beneficial options.

Knowledge is power. By arming yourself with accurate information about neuropathy, you can make informed decisions about your treatment, advocate for your well-being, and begin a journey towards improved health and quality of life.

Unveiling the Nuances of Neuropathy: Dispelling Misconceptions and Empowering Understanding

Neuropathy, a condition often shrouded in mystery, is a complex tapestry of symptoms and causes that can manifest differently in each individual. This lack of understanding can lead to misdiagnosis, delayed treatment, and misconceptions about the nature and prognosis of the condition.

So, it's crucial to dispel these misconceptions and empower individuals with accurate information to ensure they receive the most effective care and management.

While pain is a common symptom of neuropathy, it's essential to recognize that the condition can present in a variety of ways. Some individuals may experience numbness, tingling, or burning sensations without any pain. Others may have difficulty with balance, coordination, or muscle weakness.

For instance, one of our patients initially experienced numbness and tingling in their feet without pain. It wasn't until they sought further evaluation that they were diagnosed with neuropathy, highlighting the importance of recognizing the diverse symptoms of this condition.

The diverse nature of neuropathy symptoms highlights the importance of a thorough evaluation to ensure an accurate diagnosis. Early and accurate diagnosis is crucial for initiating timely treatment and preventing further nerve damage. It also allows for a personalized treatment plan that addresses the specific symptoms and underlying causes of the individual's neuropathy.

If you have concerns about your symptoms or if neuropathy continues to impact your quality of life, don't hesitate to seek a second opinion or additional testing. At

Tripp Chiropractic & Nutrition, we'll be more than happy to help you with this. It's your right to advocate for your health and ensure you receive the best possible care.

Remember, you are not alone in this journey. Resources such as patient support groups and online forums, as well as our team, can provide you with valuable support and guidance.

Why Quick Fixes Don't Work

Over-the-counter painkillers, generic supplements promising miraculous cures, and one-size-fits-all solutions often seem like attractive options for immediate relief. However, these approaches often fall short, providing only temporary respite without addressing the underlying causes of neuropathy.

A great example is the case of one of my patients, who relied heavily on pain medication for immediate relief. Initially, these medications provided some comfort, but over time, their symptoms worsened, and the reliance on painkillers grew, leading to a cycle of dependency.

Another patient sought a quick fix by trying a generic supplement advertised as a "neuropathy cure-all." Unfortunately, this approach proved worthless, with no improvement in their condition, leaving them depressed.

While quick fixes may offer a temporary reprieve from the

pain of neuropathy, they often come with significant drawbacks:

- **Cycle of dependency**: Over-reliance on pain medication can lead to addiction and tolerance, requiring higher doses for the same level of relief.
- **Potential side effects**: Painkillers and over-the-counter medications can have undesirable side effects, such as drowsiness, stomach upset, and liver or kidney damage.
- **Frustration and disappointment**: The lack of sustained improvement from quick fixes can lead to frustration, discouragement, and a loss of hope.

The path to effective neuropathy management lies in embracing sustainable solutions that address the underlying causes of the condition and promote long-term relief. This comprehensive approach may involve:

- **Lifestyle Modifications**: Again, adopting healthy habits, such as a balanced diet, regular exercise, and stress management techniques, can significantly improve nerve health and reduce symptoms.
- **Targeted Treatments**: Specific treatments may be recommended depending on the underlying cause of neuropathy, such as medications to manage blood sugar levels in diabetic neuropathy or

physical therapy to improve muscle strength and coordination.

- **Holistic Approaches**: Complementary and integrative therapies, such as acupuncture, chiropractic care, and mindfulness practices, can provide additional support and enhance overall well-being.

Navigating the complexities of neuropathy treatment requires guidance from qualified healthcare professionals. Your friendly team of neuropathy specialists at Tripp Chiropractic & Nutrition can:

- Conduct a thorough evaluation to identify the underlying cause of your peripheral neuropathy.
- Develop a personalized treatment plan tailored to your individual needs and preferences.
- Monitor your progress, make adjustments as needed, and provide ongoing support.
- Stay informed about the latest research and advancements in neuropathy treatment.

If you need help, don't hesitate to contact us by going to our website, drjasontripp.com.

As a neuropathy patient, you play an active role in managing your condition and making informed decisions about your treatment. Here are some actions you can take to empower yourself with knowledge:

- **Avoid over-reliance on instant relief**: Be cautious of solutions promising immediate cures or miracle remedies.
- **Seek sustainable treatments**: Focus on long-term management strategies that address the underlying causes of neuropathy and promote overall well-being.
- **Consult healthcare professionals**: Discuss treatment options with qualified holistic practitioners.
- **Stay informed**: Keep up-to-date with credible research and advances in neuropathy treatment through reputable sources and patient education programs.

By avoiding quick fixes, seeking professional guidance, and empowering yourself with knowledge, you can take control of your health and embark on a journey towards improved well-being.

ACTION STEP: See if your blood sugar levels are higher than the normal range. If it's high, then we must get it under control to have a good chance of reversing neuropathy symptoms.

We will test fasting blood glucose and HbA1c. If you are interested in having your blood glucose level tested scan the code below.

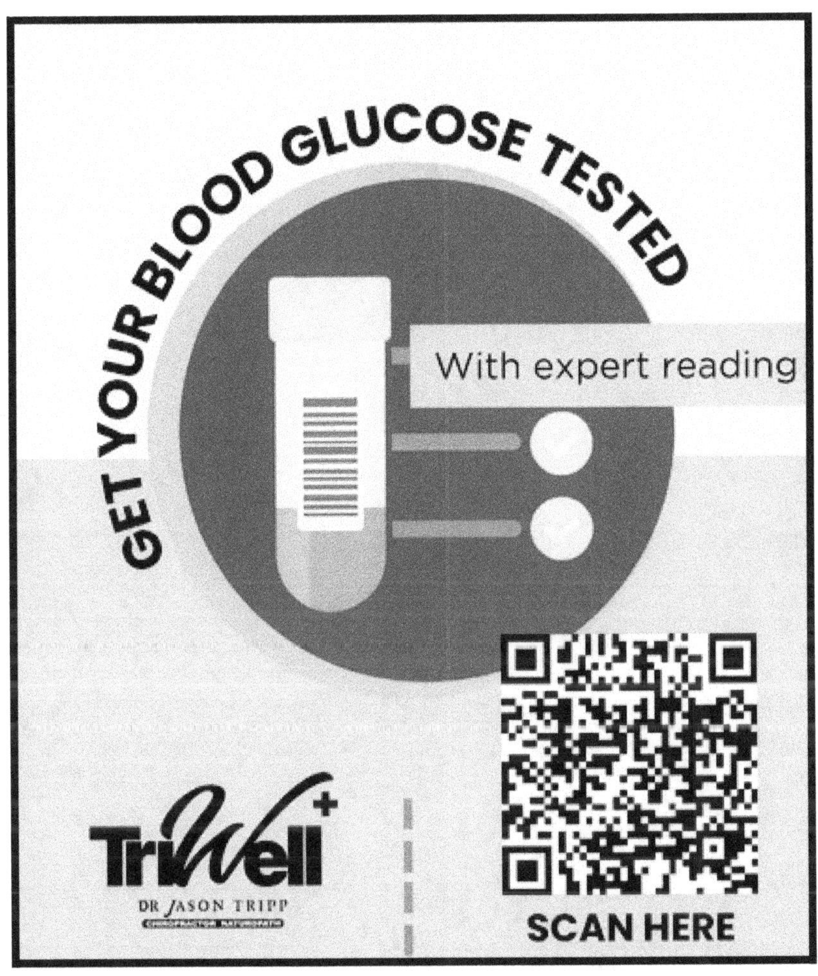

Unlock your Path to Relief Now: Dial (724) 342-2225 to speak with a Neuropathy Care Specialist Today!

4

———

UNMASKING NEUROPATHY TREATMENT MYTHS

May's Inspiring Journey: Overcoming Neuropathy and Diabetes

May came to see me for severe neuropathy in her hands and feet. She had experienced the problem 7 years ago, but it had flared up again within the past year. May was also dealing with the added complication of heel spurs. Her hands and feet felt numb, tingling, cold, and painful. As a type 2 diabetic on medication, her blood sugar levels were over 150, contributing to her condition. She had been suffering a great deal.

The neuropathy was impacting her ability to enjoy her favorite hobbies and activities. May shared, "I'm having trouble mowing, cleaning, and enjoying my hobbies." Simple tasks like walking at the mall or using a treadmill for exercise had become challenging. She used to line dance and participate in other exercises, but the neuropathy had forced her to stop. May had a goal of recovering enough to attend her granddaughter's wedding the following year.

To achieve this goal, she knew she had to get her blood sugar under control. May revealed that her A1C level was up to 11 – alarmingly high. When blood sugar remains elevated for an extended period, it slows down the healing process, especially in the fingers and toes, which was a significant contributor to her neuropathy symptoms.

We conducted our Neuropathy FREEDOM DISCOVERY VISIT exam to determine if we could help her. During this evaluation, we perform a Neuropathy Severity exam. If the exam shows that the patient has more than 85% nerve damage in the hands or feet, it is likely that little can be done to help the neuropathy, and the person would have to learn to live with it. However, if the patient has less than 85% nerve damage, we can likely provide effective treatment. When we examined May, she had less than 85% damage, but her neuropathy was still classified as severe. This meant that while we could help, the course of treatment would depend on the rest of the exam findings.

A significant portion of May's problem stemmed from her diabetes. We placed her on both the diabetes reversal protocol and the nerve regeneration protocol. May diligently followed our instructions. Within a few months, her blood sugar levels decreased, her A1C levels nearly normalized, and she felt great! May provided a wonderful testimony, stating, "I have been coming for 3 months. My hands are better, my feet are better, and my blood sugar is better."

In the world of neuropathy treatment, there's also a tangled web of myths and misconceptions that can entrap patients, leading them down paths of ineffective therapy and prolonging their suffering. As a holistic neuropathy specialist, I've witnessed firsthand the detrimental effects of these myths on so many individuals.

So, let's unmask some of these myths so you can make informed decisions about your health.

Myth: There is a one-size-fits-all cure for neuropathy.

In the quest for wellness, we often dream of a miraculous cure-all, a potion to banish every sickness. Yet, in the intricate dance of healing, neuropathy steps to a different rhythm.

Neuropathy isn't just one condition; it's a symphony of disorders, each playing its own tune of nerve damage. The variety is staggering, and that's precisely why the idea of a universal remedy is more fantasy than reality.

Picture a botanical haven, brimming with diverse flora. Each bloom and leaf unfurls, craving its own slice of sunlight and sip of water. In the same way, every neuropathy variant whispers for a custom melody of care, harmonized with the individual's unique story and the broader symphony of their health.

For instance, neuropathy caused by diabetes may require a different treatment plan than neuropathy stemming from a vitamin deficiency. Likewise, a patient with mild neuropathy may benefit from a different approach than one experiencing severe symptoms.

The mastery of neuropathy care is akin to solving a personal health puzzle, where each piece is as unique as the individual it belongs to. It's an investigative process, sifting through the annals of one's health history, the patterns of daily life, and the hidden factors that lurk beneath the surface.

With the puzzle's core piece revealed, a map to wellness can be drawn. It's a comprehensive strategy that blends the wisdom of holistic supplements, cutting edge technology, and the subtle shifts in lifestyle, all orchestrated to resonate with the patient's distinct narrative.

Myth: You just need to take medication to manage neuropathy.

While it's true that medications can provide valuable symptom relief, they're not the sole solution to this complex condition. A holistic approach encompassing lifestyle modifications alongside medication can yield far more effective and sustainable results.

Medication represents a small piece of the neuropathy puzzle, addressing the symptoms on a molecular level. However, other pieces, such as lifestyle changes, are equally crucial to complete the puzzle and achieve optimal management.

A healthy diet, rich in nutrients that support nerve function, can significantly reduce inflammation, promote nerve regeneration, and maintain overall well-being. Regular exercise, tailored to an individual's capabilities, can improve circulation, reduce nerve compression, and boost energy levels.

Stress management techniques, such as meditation, yoga, or deep breathing exercises, can help alleviate anxiety, improve sleep quality, and reduce the body's stress response, which can exacerbate neuropathy symptoms.

In some cases, lifestyle changes alone may be sufficient to manage neuropathy effectively. For instance, individuals with mild neuropathy caused by vitamin deficiencies may experience significant symptom relief by simply incorporating the missing nutrients into their diet.

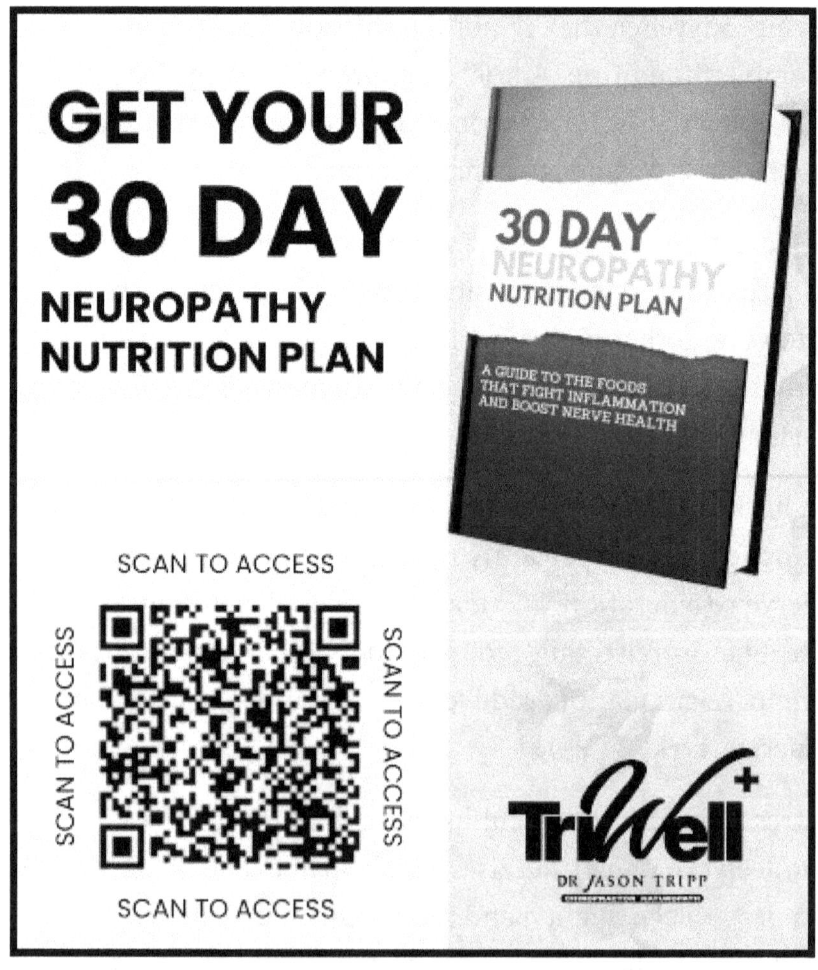

Unlock your Path to Relief Now: Dial (724) 342-2225 to speak with a Neuropathy Care Specialist Today!

Myth: Alternative therapies are not effective for neuropathy.

When managing neuropathy, the focus often revolves around conventional medical treatments and medications. However, a whole realm of alternative therapies has shown promise in alleviating symptoms, improving overall well-being, and complementing traditional treatment approaches.

Chiropractic care, focusing on the alignment of the spine and musculoskeletal system, can be beneficial for neuropathy caused by nerve compression or misalignment. Chiropractic adjustments help relieve pressure on affected nerves, improving circulation and reducing pain.

Acupuncture, a traditional Chinese medicine practice involving the insertion of thin needles into specific points on the body, has shown promising results in alleviating neuropathy pain. Studies suggest that acupuncture may induce the release of endorphins, the body's natural painkillers, while also modulating nerve activity and reducing inflammation.

Herbal supplements, such as alpha-lipoic acid, benfotiamine, and acetyl-L-carnitine, have demonstrated potential benefits in managing neuropathy symptoms. These supplements help protect nerve cells from damage, promote nerve regeneration, and reduce inflammation.

While alternative therapies can be beneficial for some neuropathy patients, it's crucial to approach them with caution and consult with a neuropathy specialist before initiating any new treatment. We can assess your needs, determine if these therapies suit you, and ensure they don't interfere with any existing medications you may be taking.

Myth: Surgery is always the best option for severe neuropathy.

In the face of severe neuropathy, surgery often emerges as a glimmer of hope, a potential solution to persistent pain and discomfort. However, it's crucial to approach surgery cautiously, understanding that it's not always the best option.

Surgery is considered only in the most extreme cases of neuropathy when other treatments, lifestyle modifications, and complementary therapies have failed to provide adequate relief.

It's important to remember that surgery is an invasive procedure with potential risks and complications, and it should only be pursued when the benefits outweigh these risks.

The decision to undergo surgery for neuropathy should not be taken lightly. It requires thoroughly discussing with your healthcare provider, carefully weighing the potential benefits and risks, considering your circumstances, and exploring all available treatment options.

In some cases, surgery can be an effective intervention, providing significant relief for individuals with severe neuropathy. For instance, surgical decompression may be considered for neuropathy caused by nerve compression, and certain surgical procedures can address specific types of nerve damage.

However, it's essential to remember that surgery is not a magic bullet. It's a tool that should be employed judiciously after exhausting other treatment options and carefully evaluating the potential benefits and risks.

Myth: There is no hope for people with neuropathy.

Neuropathy can undoubtedly present challenges and uncertainties. It's easy to feel discouraged, overwhelmed, and even hopeless when faced with persistent pain, numbness, and other symptoms that can disrupt daily life. However, there is still hope. With the right holistic treatment and a positive outlook, many people with neuropathy can live fulfilling and very productive lives.

Imagine neuropathy as a mountain to climb. It's a challenging ascent, but with the right tools and support, you can reach the summit and enjoy the view. The first step is to equip yourself with knowledge and understanding. Seek guidance from a holistic practitioner, learn about the different non-invasive, non-addictive treatment options available, and explore lifestyle changes that can support nerve health and overall well-being.

Remember, you're not alone in this journey. My team and I are more than happy to assist you. Neuropathy may be a challenge, but it's not a life sentence. With proper treatment and a positive attitude, you can reclaim your health, manage your symptoms effectively, and live a fulfilling life. Embrace hope, take control of your health, and embark on a journey towards a better tomorrow.

No Surgery Needed: Sonny's Journey from Pain to Joy

When I first started coming to Dr. Tripp, I was a real mess. I went to a couple of other doctors, and all I heard was being operated on. Well, I didn't want to be operated on because everyone I know was screwed up worse after an operation.

So I started coming here, and it was probably six weeks. I could just notice how much difference it was being on the machine, being stretched, and doing the exercises. If you do what he tells you to do, you will heal right away.

I had neuropathy down my leg, and I was dragging my leg. My disc was all messed up. And after he got done working on me, I get around great. I've never felt any better in my life. And the staff here is unbelievable. I want you people to know that if anyone tries to tell you to get an operation, please come and see Dr. Tripp before you do anything.

Sonny is living proof of the FREEDOM neuropathy program's healing power. If you're grappling with peripheral neuropathy, know that you're not alone. Reach out to Tripp Chiropractic and take the first step towards reclaiming your health and happiness.

ACTION STEP: Take our free Nerve Damage Evaluation by scanning this code:

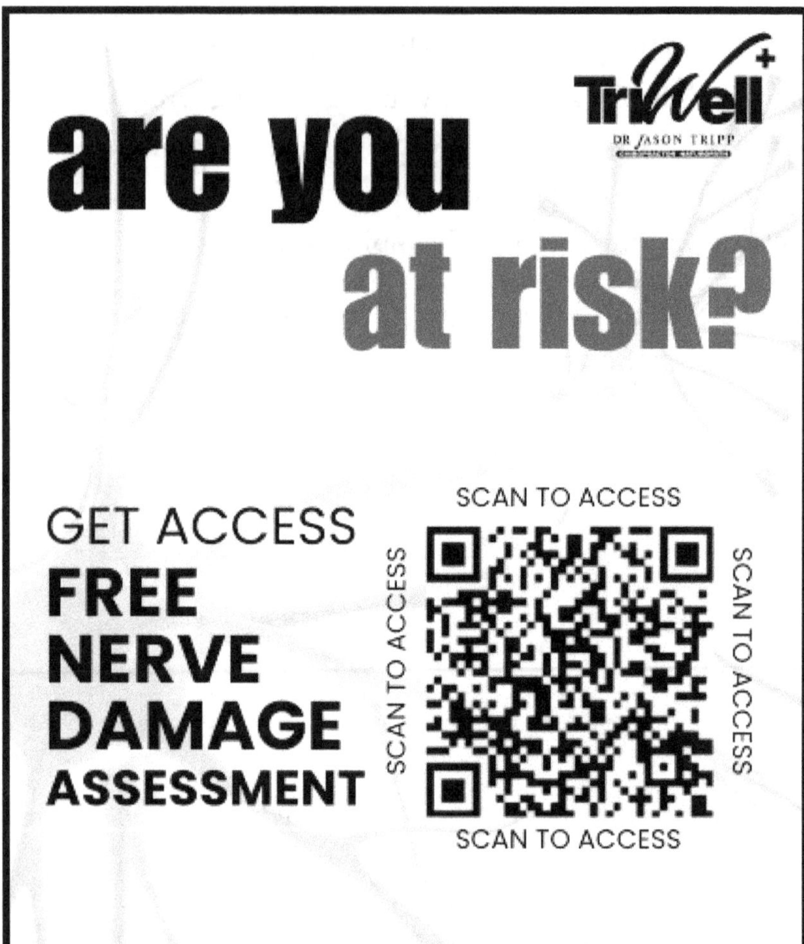

Unlock your Path to Relief Now: Dial (724) 342-2225 to speak with a Neuropathy Care Specialist Today!

5

____

REAL SECRETS TO SOLVING THE PROBLEM

Eating Your Way to Well-being: The Power of Diet in Neuropathy Management

In the landscape of neuropathy care, diet emerges not merely as fuel but as a potent ally in our quest for recovery. The act of choosing what to eat transforms into a deliberate strategy to fortify our nerves, quell the flames of inflammation, and elevate our collective health.

Consider your nerves as intricate circuitry, pulsing with life's current. They yearn for specific sustenance to maintain their dance of signals and self-repair. The B vitamins stand as pillars of this nourishment, found in the hearty fields of whole grains, the nurturing embrace of legumes, and the lush canopies of leafy greens.

Then there are the Omega-3 fatty acids, the ocean's gift, rich in the likes of salmon and tuna. These powerful compounds wield their anti-inflammatory might, soothing the sting of nerve pain and fostering a healing environment.

The chorus of science and personal stories sings in harmony—infusing our diets with these nerve-nurturing elements can usher in a renaissance of relief. Those who have walked this path speak of diminished pain, heightened sensitivity, and a retreat of numbness, a testament to the transformative power of mindful eating.

But it's not just about adding the good; it's also about reducing the bad. Processed foods, sugary drinks, and unhealthy fats can trigger inflammation in the body, exacerbating neuropathy symptoms. Opting for whole, unprocessed foods and limiting sugary indulgences can significantly impact your nerve health and overall well-being.

Staying hydrated is another crucial element of a healthy diet for neuropathy. Water transports nutrients throughout the body, including to your nerves. Proper hydration ensures your nerves function optimally and helps flush out toxins that can contribute to inflammation.

Here's a simple and delicious recipe packed with nerve-supportive nutrients.

Baked Salmon with Roasted Vegetables

Ingredients:

- 2 salmon fillets
- 1 tablespoon olive oil
- 1/2 teaspoon salt
- 1/4 teaspoon black pepper
- 1 cup Brussels sprouts, halved
- 1/2 cup red onion, sliced
- 1/2 cup sweet potato, diced
- 1/4 cup chopped fresh parsley

Instructions:

1. Preheat oven to 400°F (200°C).
2. Place salmon fillets in a baking dish. Drizzle with olive oil and season with salt and pepper.
3. Toss Brussels sprouts, onion, and sweet potato with olive oil, salt, and pepper.
4. Arrange vegetables around the salmon fillets in the baking dish.
5. Bake for 20-25 minutes, or until salmon is cooked through and vegetables are tender.
6. Garnish with fresh parsley and serve.

This recipe provides a healthy dose of protein, omega-3 fatty acids, antioxidants, and vitamins, all essential for supporting nerve health and managing neuropathy symptoms.

Remember, food is medicine. By consciously choosing nutrient-rich foods and limiting inflammatory triggers, you can actively participate in your neuropathy treatment and journey towards a healthier and happier you.

Moving Your Way to Betterment: Exercise for Neuropathy Management

When it comes to managing neuropathy, it's not just about what you eat; it's also about how you move. Regular exercise is a powerful tool in your recovery arsenal, helping you maintain muscle strength, improve coordination, reduce pain, and, ultimately, enhance your overall nerve function.

Think of your muscles as the support system for your nerves. Regular exercise strengthens these muscles, improving coordination, balance, and overall nerve function. This, in turn, helps you move with greater ease and confidence, reducing the risk of falls and injuries.

Many people with neuropathy report experiencing significant improvements in their symptoms after incorporating exercise into their routine. One patient found that a tailored exercise program helped restore their balance and reduce the frequency of falls, leading to a renewed sense of independence.

Another patient discovered that regular low-impact aerobic exercises, like swimming or walking, resulted in a noticeable decrease in their neuropathic pain, significantly improving their quality of life.

Neglecting physical activity can exacerbate neuropathy symptoms, leading to muscle weakness, reduced mobility, and even falls. However, engaging in a structured exercise program designed specifically for neuropathy management can slow the condition's progression, enhance physical capabilities, and ultimately empower you to live a more fulfilling life.

Here are some steps you can take to incorporate exercise into your neuropathy management plan:

1. **Schedule a consultation**: Meet with a holistic neuropathy specialist. They can assess your needs and develop a personalized exercise program to address your symptoms and limitations.
2. **Get moving**: Aim for at least 30 minutes of moderate-intensity exercise most days of the week. Low-impact activities like walking, swimming, or yoga are excellent for people with neuropathy.
3. **Focus on balance and strength**: Include exercises that challenge your balance and strengthen your

core muscles. These exercises can help you prevent falls and improve your overall stability.

4. **Listen to your body**: Pay attention to how your body responds to exercise. Start slowly and gradually increase the intensity and duration of your workouts as your fitness improves.

5. **Stay consistent**: The key to success is consistency. Aim to make physical activity a regular part of your routine for optimal results.

Every step counts. By incorporating physical activity into your life, you're empowering yourself to manage your neuropathy effectively, improve your physical and emotional well-being, and reclaim your zest for life.

De-stressing for better Neuropathy: Stress Management's Powerful Role

While we often focus on physical aspects of neuropathy management, the mind plays a crucial role in its relief. Chronic stress can be a hidden culprit, exacerbating symptoms and hindering your overall recovery.

The good news is that effective stress management techniques can be your secret weapon in managing neuropathy and reclaiming your well-being.

Imagine your nervous system as an exquisite orchestra, each nerve a musician poised to play in perfect harmony.

Stress, however, is the rogue trumpeter, blaring out of sync, jarring the melody of your nerves. This cacophony can swell into a crescendo of pain, numbness, and tingling —the notorious trio of neuropathy.

It's a pattern well-noted by many: stress pulls the bowstring tight, and neuropathy's arrows fly. The once tranquil concert hall of the body becomes a battleground of tension. Yet, there is hope in the form of stress-busting maestros like meditation and deep breathing. These practices strike a chord of balance, quieting the mind's turmoil and the body's unrest.

Those who master these techniques often share tales of transformation—of symptoms softened and a sense of command restored. They become conductors of their own well-being.

In the same vein, yoga emerges as a kindred spirit, a practice that marries movement with the breath's quiet rhythm. It's a dance that lulls the stress hormones to sleep and awakens a state of serenity. The result? A life's symphony played softer, sleep that comes easier, and a view of life through a lens of optimism.

Ignoring the impact of stress on neuropathy can be detrimental to your physical and emotional well-being. However, adopting effective stress management strategies can make a world of difference. Here are some steps you can take:

1. **Identify your stress triggers**: Recognizing what triggers your stress response is the first step toward managing it. Take time to reflect on situations or events that typically cause you to feel anxious or overwhelmed.

2. **Embrace relaxation techniques**: Meditation, deep breathing, and yoga are powerful tools for calming the mind and body. Find techniques that resonate with you and incorporate them into your daily routine.

3. **Practice mindfulness**: Pay attention to the present moment without judgment. Mindfulness can help you become more aware of your thoughts and emotions and respond to stress in a more mindful and healthy way.

Even simple breathing exercises can have a significant impact on stress levels. Here's one you can try right now.

4-7-8 Breathing Technique

1. Close your mouth and inhale slowly through your nose for a count of 4.
2. Hold your breath for a count of 7.
3. Exhale slowly through your mouth for a count of 8.
4. Repeat this cycle several times until you feel a sense of calm and relaxation.

Stress management is not a one-time fix; it's an ongoing process. By consciously managing your stress, you can create a more peaceful environment for your nervous system to heal and thrive. So embrace stress management techniques as powerful allies in your journey towards neuropathy relief and overall well-being.

Beyond Medications: Exploring Integrative Medicine for Neuropathy Relief

Medication is a cornerstone in the fortress against neuropathy, but it's not the sole guardian. Integrative medicine is like the skilled artisan who weaves traditional methods with the threads of alternative wisdom to craft a tapestry of care that envelops your entire being.

Imagine your health as a mosaic, intricate and multifaceted. The pieces laid by conventional medicine shine brightly, yet it's the stones placed by integrative practices that fill the gaps, creating a portrait of health that's complete and truly yours. This artful blend allows us to delve deep, targeting the very roots of neuropathy and nurturing you back to a state of harmony.

Many patients have found significant relief by incorporating integrative therapies alongside their medication regimen. Some individuals have experienced reduced pain and improved nerve function after integrating acupuncture into their treatment plan. Others have discovered that herbal supplements offer more effective symptom management when combined with chiropractic care than supplements alone.

Integrative approaches require more coordination and effort than a simple pill, but the benefits are worth it. By addressing your neuropathy from multiple angles, you can often achieve better symptom control and improve your overall health and well-being. This holistic approach can also help reduce your reliance on medications and potentially minimize their side effects.

Here are some steps you can take to explore the potential of integrative medicine for neuropathy:

1. **Research complementary therapies**: Learn more about acupuncture, massage therapy, chiropractic care, herbal supplements, and other alternative approaches that may complement your current treatment plan.
2. **Open communication with your healthcare provider**: Discuss your interest in integrative medicine and explore options that may suit you.
3. **Monitor your response**: Pay close attention to how your body reacts to each integrative therapy and observe any changes in your neuropathy symptoms.

4. **Join my peripheral neuropathy workshop**: This workshop will delve into the FREEDOM method and discuss the possibility of integrating alternative therapies into your current treatment plan. Click here to register today or visit https://www.neradreviveprogram.com/workshop-registration-page-tripp, and take the first step towards a more holistic approach to neuropathy management.

By embracing a comprehensive approach that combines conventional medicine with the wisdom of integrative medicine, you can unlock a new level of healing and reclaim a life of vibrant health and well-being.

Suzanne's Success Story

I really appreciate what Dr. Tripp has done for me. When I first went to him, I was 69 pounds heavier on my left side, and I had trouble walking up the stairs. I could hardly lift my leg. After multiple adjustments, I was able to climb stairs normally. I've had neck problems, but my neck is improving. I also have neuropathy in my feet, and they are getting much better through adjustments and therapy. This doctor knows what he's doing! Thank you so much, Dr. Tripp!

ACTION STEP: Scan the code below to download our 25 Anti-Inflammatory Recipes Guide.

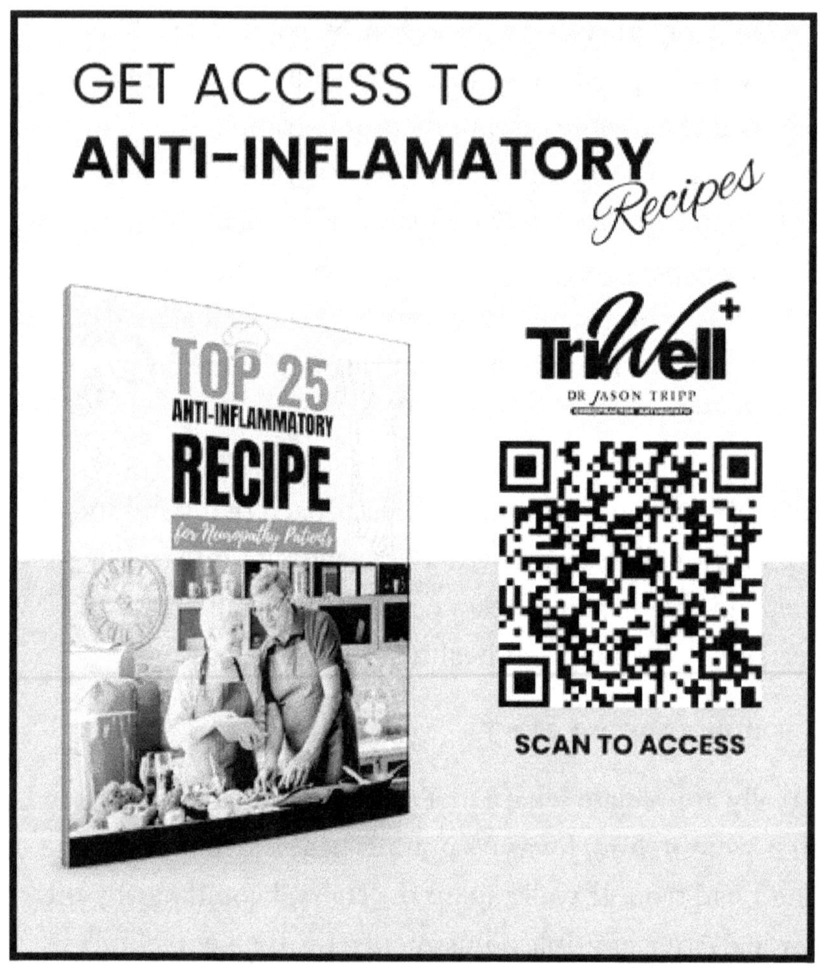

Unlock your Path to Relief Now: Dial (724) 342-2225 to speak with a Neuropathy Care Specialist Today!

6

THE FREEDOM METHOD: YOUR ROADMAP TO RECLAIMING YOUR LIFE FROM NEUROPATHY

As a holistic doctor specializing in peripheral neuropathy, I've witnessed firsthand the frustration and limitations this condition can impose on people's lives. That's why I'm excited to share the TriWell Nerve F.R.E.E.D.O.M. Method, a unique approach designed to help you reclaim your health and well-being.

Each letter in F.R.E.E.D.O.M. represents a crucial step in your recovery journey:

F - Find Root Cause

R - Restore Normal Function

E - Eliminate Root Cause

E - Elevate Your Health

D - Discover Wellness

O - Optimal Nutrition

M - Maintain Health Wellness Lifestyle

Let's explore each aspect of the FREEDOM neuropathy method in greater detail so you can understand why it's the key to unlocking your health and well-being.

F - Find Root Cause

Neuropathy is a symptom, not a disease itself. It's like the red warning light on your car's dashboard – it tells you something is wrong, but it doesn't tell you what. Our mission in this first phase is to identify the underlying issue triggering your neuropathy.

Here's why this is so critical:

- **Targeted Treatment**: Understanding the root cause allows us to tailor a treatment plan specifically for you. A one-size-fits-all approach simply doesn't work for neuropathy.
- **Long-Term Relief**: By addressing the underlying cause, we can prevent the neuropathy from progressing and promote lasting healing. Masking symptoms with medication might offer temporary relief, but it doesn't fix the problem.

- **Preventing Recurrence**: Knowing the root cause empowers you to make lifestyle changes or take preventive measures to minimize the risk of future flare-ups.

During this initial phase, we'll dive into your medical history, discuss your current symptoms in detail, and perform a thorough physical examination. Specialized testing may also be necessary depending on your individual case. This comprehensive investigation allows us to uncover potential culprits like vitamin deficiencies, hidden infections, autoimmune conditions, or even chronic inflammation.

Remember, finding the root cause is the foundation for our entire FREEDOM program. By taking the time to identify the culprit behind your neuropathy, we lay the groundwork for a targeted, effective treatment plan that can truly set you free from pain and reclaim your quality of life.

R - Restore Normal Function

Imagine your peripheral nerves as the body's information superhighway. When these nerves are damaged due to neuropathy, the messages traveling between your brain and body become disrupted. This can manifest in a variety of ways, from burning pain and tingling to numbness and weakness. Our goal in this phase is to help your body restore normal function to these vital pathways.

Here's how we'll achieve this:

- **Chiropractic Care**: Targeted chiropractic adjustments can help improve nerve communication by ensuring proper spinal alignment and reducing inflammation around the nerve roots. Think of it as gently detangling the wires in your body's communication network.
- **Physical Therapy**: Specific exercises can help improve muscle strength, coordination, and balance, all of which are often compromised by neuropathy. Regaining control over your movements not only boosts confidence but also helps retrain the brain-body connection.
- **Other Therapies**: Depending on your individual needs, we may incorporate additional therapies like therapeutic ultrasound, electrical stimulation, or even acupuncture to promote nerve healing and pain reduction.

It's important to remember that your body is capable of remarkable healing. By addressing the root cause and implementing these targeted therapies, we can create an environment that optimizes your body's natural ability to repair and regenerate damaged nerves.

This phase of Restoring Normal Function goes beyond simply managing pain. It's about empowering you to regain control and reclaim your life. As nerve function improves, you'll likely experience a decrease in pain, but more importantly, you'll be able to move with greater ease, participate in activities you once enjoyed, and experience a renewed sense of freedom and well-being.

E - Eliminate Root Cause

Think of this stage as the counteroffensive in our battle against neuropathy. Armed with the knowledge of the root cause, we can now develop a targeted strategy to neutralize the enemy and prevent it from causing further damage.

Here's how eliminating the root cause might look depending on the culprit:

- **Nutritional Deficiencies**: If vitamin deficiencies are contributing to your neuropathy, we'll develop a personalized supplement plan to address those specific shortfalls. A balanced diet rich in essential nutrients is also crucial for optimal nerve health.
- **Chronic Inflammation**: If underlying inflammation is the culprit, we'll explore dietary modifications, anti-inflammatory supplements, and other natural approaches to reduce inflammation throughout the body.

- **Autoimmune Conditions**: In cases where an autoimmune disorder is at play, we'll work closely with your primary physician to develop a treatment plan that manages the underlying condition and protects your nerves from further damage.

Eliminating the root cause often extends beyond simply addressing a medical condition. It may also involve making some key lifestyle modifications. For example, if diabetes is a contributing factor, we'll discuss strategies for blood sugar control through diet, exercise, and potentially medication if needed.

Remember, these lifestyle changes are not punishments; they're powerful tools for taking charge of your health and preventing future neuropathy flare-ups. We'll work together to create a sustainable plan that fits your unique needs and preferences.

E - Elevate Your Health

This phase is all about empowering your body's natural healing mechanisms and creating an optimal environment for nerve repair and regeneration.

Neuropathy thrives in a stressed and imbalanced body. By elevating your overall health, we can significantly improve your chances of achieving lasting relief and preventing future flare-ups. Here's how we'll achieve this:

- **Nutritional Optimization**: We'll explore the world of nutrition, and examine how specific foods and dietary patterns can promote nerve health. This may involve incorporating anti-inflammatory foods, essential supplements, and antioxidants into your diet.
- **Stress Management**: Chronic stress wreaks havoc on your entire system, including your nerves. We'll explore stress-reduction techniques like meditation, yoga, or deep breathing exercises to help you manage stress effectively.
- **Quality Sleep**: Sleep is essential for nerve repair and overall well-being. We'll discuss strategies for improving your sleep hygiene and achieving restorative sleep each night.
- **Regular Exercise**: Physical activity is a powerful tool for managing neuropathy pain and promoting nerve health. We'll develop a safe and effective exercise program tailored to your fitness level and capabilities.

The FREEDOM method emphasizes a holistic approach to healing neuropathy. We're not just treating your nerves; we're addressing your entire well-being. By optimizing your nutrition, managing stress, prioritizing sleep, and incorporating regular exercise, we create a powerful foundation for your body's natural healing processes to kick in.

Elevating your health isn't just about symptom relief; it's about creating a lifestyle that promotes long-term vitality and overall well-being. As you make these positive changes, you'll likely experience not only a reduction in neuropathy symptoms but also increased energy levels, improved mood, and a stronger, more resilient body.

D - Discover Wellness

Now, it's time to discover wellness by exploring the world of complementary therapies that can further enhance your healing journey and improve your quality of life.

While traditional medical approaches are essential for treating neuropathy, complementary therapies can offer a wealth of benefits. Here's how some of these therapies can support your healing:

- **Massage Therapy**: Therapeutic massage can promote relaxation, reduce muscle tension, and improve circulation, all of which can contribute to pain relief and overall well-being.
- **Mind-Body Techniques**: Meditation, yoga, and mindfulness practices can help manage stress,

improve sleep quality, and promote a sense of calm, all of which can be beneficial for neuropathy patients.

It's important to remember that complementary therapies are not a one-size-fits-all solution. We'll work together to explore different options and find the ones that resonate most with you and best complement your overall treatment plan.

The Power of Self-Care

Discovering wellness is also about embracing self-care practices that nurture your body, mind, and spirit. This might involve spending time in nature, engaging in hobbies you enjoy, or simply prioritizing activities that bring you joy and a sense of peace.

By incorporating these complementary therapies and self-care practices into your routine, you'll discover a powerful toolbox for managing your neuropathy and enhancing your overall well-being.

O - Optimal Nutrition

You are what you eat, and the food you choose can significantly impact your nerve health and overall healing potential. In this phase, we'll explore how to leverage the power of food to nourish your nerves and support your body's natural repair mechanisms.

Think of food as medicine: By incorporating specific nutrients and dietary patterns, we can create an internal environment that promotes nerve healing and reduces inflammation, a major contributor to neuropathy pain. Here's how optimal nutrition can make a difference:

- **Antioxidant Powerhouse**: Antioxidants combat harmful free radicals that damage cells, including nerve cells. We'll focus on incorporating fruits, vegetables, and whole grains rich in antioxidants into your diet.
- **Essential Fatty Acids**: Omega-3 fatty acids play a crucial role in nerve health and function. Fatty fish, flaxseeds, and walnuts are excellent sources of these essential fats.
- **B Vitamin Bonanza**: B vitamins are vital for nerve function. We'll ensure your diet includes foods rich in B vitamins, such as leafy greens, legumes, and nuts.
- **Staying Hydrated**: Dehydration can worsen neuropathy symptoms. Drinking plenty of water is essential for optimal nerve function and overall health.

Optimal nutrition goes beyond simply following a specific diet. It's also about understanding how certain foods might affect your individual neuropathy symptoms. We'll work together to identify any potential food triggers that might exacerbate your pain and create a personalized eating plan that works best for you.

Remember, the goal is to create healthy eating habits that you can maintain for the long term. We'll focus on making gradual, sustainable changes that fit your lifestyle and preferences. Small tweaks, like incorporating more vegetables into your meals or swapping sugary drinks for water, can make a big difference in your overall health and nerve function.

By prioritizing optimal nutrition, you're not just feeding your body; you're providing the essential building blocks your nerves need to heal and regenerate.

M - Maintain Health Wellness Lifestyle

We've reached a pivotal point in your neuropathy journey. Throughout the TriWell Nerve FREEDOM Program, we've identified the root cause, restored nerve function, eliminated the root cause, addressed your overall health, explored complementary therapies, and harnessed the power of optimal nutrition. Now, it's time to solidify these positive changes and make them a permanent part of your life with M – Maintain Health & Wellness Lifestyle.

Think of this stage as a roadmap for long-term success. Neuropathy is a chronic condition, but by maintaining healthy habits, you can significantly reduce the risk of flare-ups and experience lasting relief. Here's how we'll achieve this:

- **Habit Formation**: We'll work together to develop healthy habits that become an automatic part of your daily routine. This might involve scheduling regular exercise sessions, planning healthy meals in advance, or incorporating stress-management techniques into your day.
- **Building Support Systems**: A strong support system is crucial for long-term success. We'll discuss ways to involve your family and friends in your health journey and create a network of encouragement and accountability.
- **Staying Motivated**: Maintaining healthy habits can be challenging. We'll explore strategies for staying motivated, such as setting realistic goals, celebrating your progress, and finding ways to make healthy choices enjoyable.
- **Regular Check-Ins**: Scheduling regular chiropractic appointments allows us to monitor your progress, address any new concerns, and fine-tune your treatment plan as needed.

Maintaining a healthy lifestyle isn't just about managing neuropathy; it's about preventing future flare-ups and promoting overall well-being. By continuing these healthy habits, you're empowering your body to stay strong and resilient, reducing the risk of future nerve damage.

We'll be here to support you every step of the way, offering guidance, encouragement, and ongoing chiropractic care to ensure you stay on the path to lasting freedom from neuropathy.

How Galen Reclaimed His Health and Happiness with Tripp Chiropractic & Nutrition

Galen was suffering from chronic pain and numbness that affected his quality of life. He had trouble walking, sitting, sleeping, and doing the things he loved. He felt hopeless and frustrated with his condition. He had tried different treatments, but nothing seemed to work.

That's when he decided to give Tripp Chiropractic & Nutrition a try. He was impressed by our holistic approach and personalized care. He learned how to improve his posture, nutrition, and lifestyle habits. He received gentle and effective adjustments that relieved his pain and restored his mobility.

After just a month of treatment, Galen felt like a new person. He was able to move freely and comfortably. He could enjoy his hobbies and activities again. He felt more energetic, confident, and happy. He said he felt 90% better than he did before. He was amazed by the results and grateful for our help.

Galen is one of the many success stories of Tripp Chiropractic & Nutrition. If you are looking for a natural and lasting solution to your health problems, contact us today and see how we can help you.

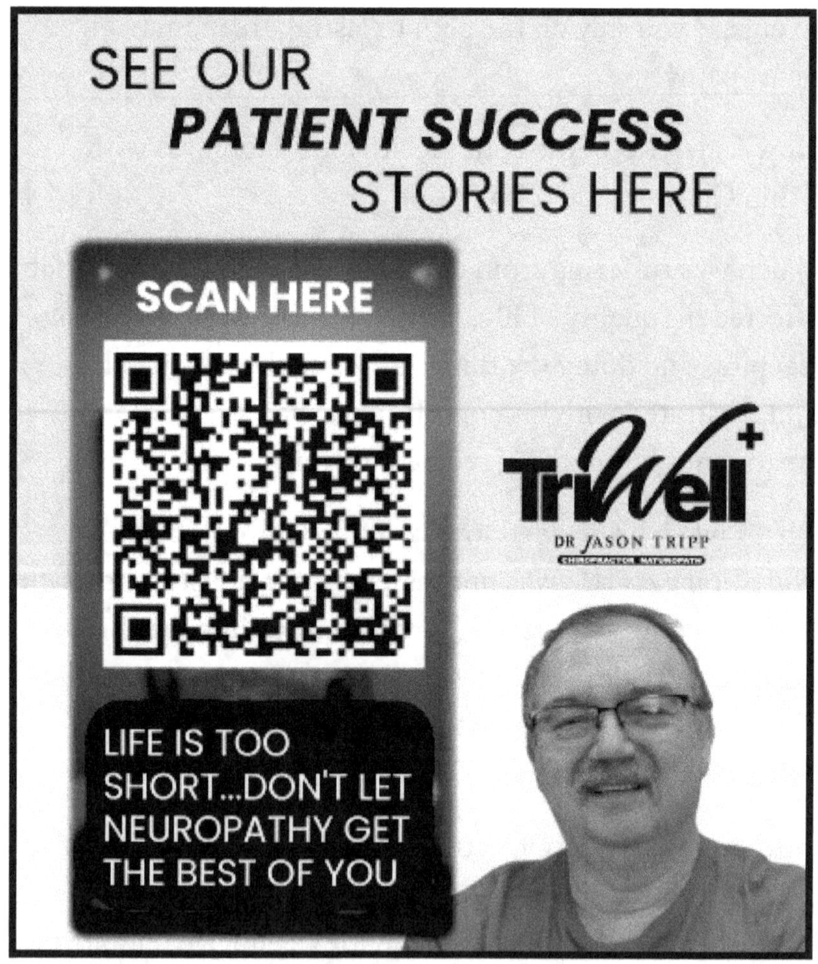

Unlock your Path to Relief Now: Dial (724) 342-2225 to speak with a Neuropathy Care Specialist Today!

7

———

YOUR NERVOUS SYSTEM: THE BODY'S MASTER CONDUCTOR

The intricate workings of your nervous system are truly a marvel. Imagine your body as a complex orchestra, each part playing a vital role in the symphony of life. Now, picture the nervous system as the conductor, wielding the baton and ensuring everything runs smoothly. From the delicate dance of your muscles to the rhythmic thrum of your heart, nerves act as lightning-fast messengers, coordinating every function. But what happens when this maestro of the body faces a serious challenge? What if multiple instruments are out of tune, creating a cacophony instead of a harmonious melody?

This is the situation Alexa found herself in. Diagnosed with both multiple sclerosis and epilepsy, she also experienced the agonizing effects of neuropathy, a constant burning and tingling in her leg that impacted every aspect of her

97

life. It would have been easy to surrender to these overwhelming health challenges. But Alexa's story isn't one of defeat; it's a powerful testament to the body's remarkable capacity for healing.

Triumph Over Multiple Challenges

It's stories like Alexa's that remind me why I dedicated my life to helping people overcome seemingly insurmountable health challenges. Alexa came to us facing a double whammy: multiple sclerosis (MS), which she'd been battling for 32 years, and epilepsy, a companion for 47 years. On top of that, her MS had relapsed in 2017, leaving her with debilitating neuropathy in her left leg.

The constant burning, pins-and-needles sensation was relentless, a torment that permeated every aspect of her life. But Alexa was determined to find relief. She committed fully to both our chiropractic and nutrition programs, the cornerstones of the FREEDOM method. What happened next was nothing short of remarkable. In just four weeks, her neuropathy vanished! But that was just the beginning. She continued the programs, lost 45 pounds, and achieved full remission from her MS.

Witnessing Alexa's transformation firsthand was deeply moving. She not only reclaimed her health but also discovered a new passion for helping others. Today, she's a valued member of our staff, sharing her inspiring story and guiding others on their own healing journeys. Alexa's success is a testament to the power of a holistic approach, the unwavering human spirit, and the potential for profound healing that lies within each of us.

Peripheral neuropathy disrupts this beautiful harmony. Think of it like frayed cables causing static in the communication lines. Those once-crisp signals carrying messages to your body now flicker and sputter, leading to the tingling, burning, or numbness you experience in your feet, legs, or hands. But the impact of neuropathy goes far deeper.

Unreliable nerve signals can throw off your balance, making even a simple walk feel like a tightrope act. They can wreak havoc on your digestion, leading to uncomfortable bloating or constipation. Even restful sleep becomes a distant memory as those misfiring signals keep you tossing and turning through the night.

Here's the empowering truth: your body is a magnificent healer, and that extends to your nervous system. While neuropathy may seem daunting, the FREEDOM approach focuses on unlocking your body's inherent ability to mend itself. We'll create an environment conducive to nerve regeneration, allowing function to gradually return and the music of your body to play its beautiful song once more.

Understanding Your Nervous System: Friend or Foe in Neuropathy?

Have you ever wondered how a simple touch, a delicious taste, or even a spontaneous thought translates into action within your body? The answer lies in your amazing nervous system, and understanding its workings can shed light on how neuropathy disrupts this intricate network.

Think of your nervous system as a vast communication hub. It has two key players:

- **Central Nervous System (CNS)**: This is your body's command center, encompassing your brain and spinal cord. It acts as the processing unit, interpreting information, generating thoughts and emotions, and sending instructions throughout the body.
- **Peripheral Nervous System (PNS)**: Imagine the PNS as a complex web of communication cables branching out from your spinal cord. These cables connect your CNS to every organ, muscle, and even the tiniest tissue. They're responsible for relaying sensations like touch and temperature, controlling your movements, and even influencing automatic functions like your heart rate. This is precisely the system that neuropathy primarily targets.

Let's take a closer look at the individual "cables" within this network – the nerves themselves. Each nerve is like a tiny, insulated wire. The core wire, carrying the message, is called the axon. Surrounding this core is a crucial protective layer known as the myelin sheath. Think of it like the rubber coating safeguarding an electrical wire.

In neuropathy, the damage can occur to both the axon and the myelin sheath. If the protective sheath is compromised, the messages get scrambled, resulting in pain. In other cases, the core wire itself might be affected, leading to numbness. These damaged nerves are the culprits behind the frustrating symptoms you experience with neuropathy.

The Plot Twist: How Nerves Get Hijacked in Neuropathy

We've talked about the amazing communication network that is your nervous system. But what happens when this finely tuned system goes awry? That's where neuropathy enters the picture, and it can manifest in a few different ways:

- **Peripheral Neuropathy**: This is our area of expertise. It's when the nerves in your extremities – your hands, feet, legs, and sometimes even arms – become compromised. This is the culprit behind the frustrating tingling, burning, and numbness you might be experiencing.

- **Autonomic Neuropathy**: This less common type affects the nerves that control your body's "automatic functions" like digestion, heart rate, and blood pressure. While less frequent, it's important to be aware of its potential impact.

So, how does this nerve hijacking happen? It's rarely a single villain at play. Instead, neuropathy often results from a combination of factors creating a domino effect of damage. Let's explore some of the biggest culprits:

- **Unstable Blood Sugar**: Wild swings in blood sugar wreak havoc on your entire body, and your nerves are no exception.
- **Chronic Inflammation**: Imagine this as a constant low-grade fire burning throughout your body. Nerves are particularly vulnerable to this inflammatory damage.
- **Nutritional Deficiencies**: Your nerves, like any hardworking team, need specific vitamins and minerals to function optimally and repair themselves. When your diet lacks these essential nutrients, your nerve health suffers.
- **Underlying Medical Conditions**: Diabetes is a well-known risk factor, but neuropathy can also be a companion to autoimmune disorders, thyroid problems, and even past infections or exposure to

toxins.

The key takeaway? To truly conquer neuropathy, we need to go beyond simply masking the symptoms. We need to become detectives, uncovering the root causes that are fueling the problem.

The Body's Built-in Repair Kit: Unleashing Your Nerve Healing Potential

Here's the incredibly good news: Your body isn't a static machine. It has a remarkable ability to heal, and that includes your nerves. This is where a concept called neuroplasticity comes in. Neuroplasticity means your brain and nerves can change, adapt, and form new connections, essentially rewiring themselves to overcome damage – a powerful tool in your FREEDOM toolbox.

While this doesn't happen overnight, it's the foundation of true healing for neuropathy. So, how do we support this natural healing process? Let's break it down:

- **Specific Nutrients**: Your nerves are hungry for B vitamins, magnesium, and other key nutrients. These act as building blocks for repair and protect against further damage.
- **Lifestyle Adjustments**: Simple lifestyle adjustments like getting restorative sleep, managing stress, and incorporating the right types

of movement all work together to reduce inflammation and create a better environment for your nerves to heal.

- **The FREEDOM Approach**: Our therapies are designed to directly stimulate nerve regeneration, increase blood flow to damaged areas, and calm that "fire" of inflammation. Combined with targeted nutrition and those lifestyle shifts, this creates a powerful synergy for healing.

It's important to remember that healing takes time and consistency. But by understanding and actively supporting your body's innate healing mechanisms, you unlock the potential for real, lasting improvement in your neuropathy.

The Mind-Body Link: Your Untapped Resource for Nerve Restoration

We often think of healing in purely physical terms, but when it comes to neuropathy, we can't ignore the mind-body connection. Let's dive into why this matters.

Stress – The Hidden Enemy

When you're constantly stressed, your body is in a chronic "fight or flight" mode. This floods your system with stress hormones, worsens inflammation, and ultimately makes your neuropathy symptoms flare up. Plus, it keeps you in a state where healing simply can't be a priority.

Stress Relief: Key to Healing

Finding ways to manage stress isn't just about feeling better in the moment, it's about unlocking your body's ability to heal. Here are some techniques well-suited for those with neuropathy:

- **Mindfulness Practices**: Simple focusing exercises, like noticing your breath for a few minutes, can pull you into the present and calm a racing mind. Mindfulness practices like focusing on your breath can create a sense of calm, allowing your body to redirect its energy towards healing and nerve regeneration.
- **Gentle Movement**: Yoga, Tai Chi, or simply mindful walking can be great ways to release tension and improve circulation.
- **Guided Relaxation**: There are many apps or audio recordings offering guided meditations, helping you shift into a more relaxed state.

The key is finding what works for you. Even 5-10 minutes of these practices daily can make a significant difference over time.

Positivity: Your Powerful Ally in Nerve Restoration

You might think a positive mindset is just feel-good fluff, but when it comes to neuropathy, it's much more powerful than that.

The Self-Fulfilling Prophecy

If you believe your neuropathy has you trapped, and that it will only get worse, those thoughts become a roadblock to progress. However, when you cultivate the belief that healing IS possible, you're more likely to embrace the FREEDOM program wholeheartedly.

Mind Over Matter

A positive mindset isn't a magic bullet, but it's a powerful tool. It reduces stress (a known roadblock to healing), increases motivation, and empowers you to face challenges with greater resilience.

Hope Is Fuel

The healing journey can be long. Belief in your body's ability to improve and faith in the FREEDOM process can make all the difference in staying committed, even when progress feels slow. It's important to be honest about the challenges, but don't let fear or past disappointments steal your hope. Empower yourself by focusing on the potential for a better tomorrow.

By now, you have a much deeper understanding of how your amazing nervous system works and the ways that neuropathy disrupts its delicate balance. This knowledge isn't just about knowing the facts; it's about empowerment. The more you understand, the clearer it becomes that you're not just a victim of this condition; you're an active participant in your healing journey.

FREEDOM is designed to be a partnership. It honors the complexity of neuropathy by addressing not just the physical damage, but the mental, emotional, and lifestyle factors that so greatly impact your overall nervous system health.

Think of it this way: If your nerves are that intricate communication network, we're providing the tools to repair the wires, boost the signal quality, and even teach your brain and body healthier communication patterns. This multi-pronged approach is what sets FREEDOM apart, offering true holistic healing and the best chance of lasting relief from neuropathy.

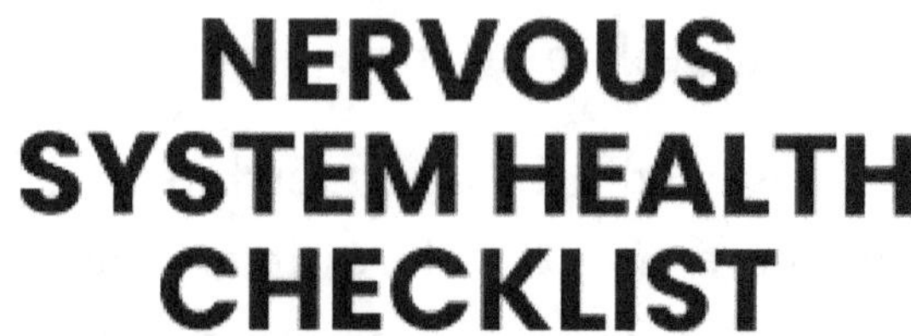

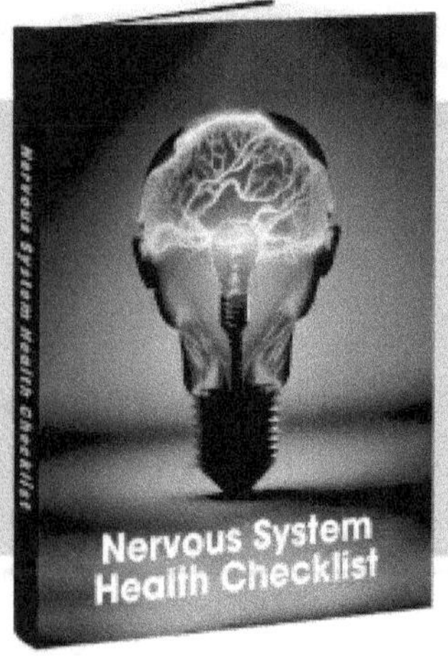

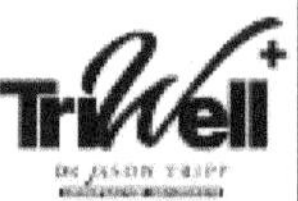

Unlock your Path to Relief Now: Dial (724) 342-2225 to speak with a Neuropathy Care Specialist Today!

8

———

WHEN STATINS HURT MORE THAN THEY HELP: A CLOSER LOOK AT NERVE DAMAGE

If you're among the millions taking statins to lower cholesterol, it's vital to understand the implications, especially if you're battling neuropathy. As one of the most commonly prescribed medications globally, statins deserve a closer look for anyone managing chronic conditions.

For decades, the message on cholesterol has been clear-cut: high cholesterol is the enemy, and aggressive lowering is the solution. But recent research paints a more nuanced picture, prompting the question – are statin benefits always worth the potential drawbacks?

This is particularly relevant for those with neuropathy. Studies reveal a concerning link between statin use and an increased risk of developing neuropathy, or a worsening of existing symptoms. Unfortunately, many patients (and even some healthcare providers) remain unaware of this potential side effect. This chapter empowers you with the knowledge to make informed decisions about your health.

The Statin Conundrum: Balancing Cholesterol with Nerve Health

Let's examine how statins function within your body and why, despite their intended benefit, they might have unintended consequences.

Statins: Curbing Cholesterol Production

Your liver is the body's cholesterol-manufacturing plant. Statins act like a dimmer switch, slowing down this production line – seemingly a good solution for high cholesterol. However, the picture isn't black and white.

The CoQ10 Connection

The liver doesn't just churn out cholesterol; it also produces CoQ10, a vital cellular fuel for energy production in every cell. Imagine CoQ10 as the spark plugs in your cellular power plants. Here's the hitch: statins block the pathway that creates CoQ10, often leading to depleted CoQ10 levels alongside lower cholesterol.

Why CoQ10 Matters for Nerves

Your nerves and muscles are energy guzzlers. Depleting

their CoQ10 fuel source can trigger symptoms eerily similar to neuropathy – weakness, pain, fatigue, and more.

Beyond Neuropathy: A Wider Net of Side Effects

The conversation on statins wouldn't be complete without acknowledging the broader spectrum of side effects reported by users. These include muscle aches, difficulty concentrating (brain fog), blood sugar imbalances, and even a potential increased risk for Parkinson's and liver damage. While some might dismiss these as minor, they significantly impact quality of life, especially when dealing with a condition like neuropathy.

Statins and Neuropathy: Navigating the Research with Caution

Unfortunately, research paints a clear picture: statins and neuropathy have a closer connection than many patients realize. Let's explore the evidence and understand why this necessitates careful consideration when making treatment decisions.

Increased Vulnerability: Who's Most at Risk?

Certain factors elevate the risk of statin-induced neuropathy:

- **Pre-existing Neuropathy or Diabetes**: If your

nerves are already compromised, statins can further weaken them.

- **Age**: As we age, our bodies become less efficient at processing medications, increasing the likelihood of side effects.
- **Polypharmacy**: Interactions between statins and other medications can raise complication risks.
- **Vitamin D Deficiency**: Low Vitamin D levels might worsen the nerve-damaging effects of statins.

The Misdiagnosis Trap

Imagine experiencing worsening neuropathy symptoms – increased burning, weakness, and walking difficulty – while taking a statin. Often, the assumption (even by some doctors) is that the neuropathy itself is simply progressing. This can lead to:

- **Increased Statin Dosage**: The thought process goes: "If high cholesterol is the culprit, and levels aren't dropping enough, we need a higher dose." Unfortunately, this can significantly worsen side effects.
- **Additional Medications**: Doctors might prescribe medications specifically for nerve pain, not considering the statin as a potential contributor.
- **Unnecessary Anxiety**: The belief that the condition is worsening can add significant mental

and emotional stress on top of the physical discomfort.

The situation becomes even trickier because some patients with statin-induced neuropathy might experience initial improvement as cholesterol levels decrease. This can create a false sense of security, masking the long-term nerve damage caused by the statin.

The crucial message? If you're on a statin and experience ANY change in your neuropathy symptoms – positive or negative – discuss it thoroughly with your doctor. Don't simply assume every setback signifies disease progression.

The good news is that there are other paths to healing, paths that work with your body's natural ability to repair and regenerate. Jill's experience is a perfect example. She came to us with her feet in terrible condition due to neuropathy, a common struggle for individuals battling statin-induced nerve damage. After just two months on the FREEDOM program, she reported significant improvement, saying her feet are 'a lot better now'. This highlights that even when neuropathy feels overwhelming, there is hope for recovery through natural, holistic methods.

Natural Strategies for Heart Health: Protecting Your Body From the Inside Out

Natural approaches offer a powerful, multifaceted way to support your cardiovascular system AND address the very factors that accelerate neuropathy progression.

Beyond Cholesterol: Addressing the Root Causes

Think of inflammation as a fire smoldering inside your blood vessels. Over time, this fire damages the delicate lining, making it rough and prone to accumulating debris. This is where cholesterol has its chance to build up, forming dangerous plaques that can lead to heart attack or stroke. Statins address high cholesterol numbers, but they don't extinguish the underlying fire.

Oxidative damage is another culprit. Imagine all your cells, including those lining your blood vessels, constantly producing 'exhaust fumes' from energy production. Antioxidants act as your body's air filtration system, neutralizing these fumes. When inflammation and an unhealthy lifestyle overload this system, it's like 'rusting' your blood vessels from the inside out.

Why does this matter for neuropathy? Your nerves are especially vulnerable to both inflammation and oxidative damage. The very things that threaten your heart health are also contributing to the breakdown of your nerves. By tackling these root issues, you're not just protecting your heart – you're safeguarding your entire body, especially those vulnerable nerves.

Lifestyle as Medicine: Your Body's Natural Defense System

Let's explore the immense power of lifestyle modifications in protecting your heart and nerves. Prioritize an anti-inflammatory diet. Ditch processed foods and fill your plate with vibrant, whole foods. Think of those colorful fruits and vegetables as an army of antioxidants, safeguarding your blood vessels and nerves. It's also crucial to choose foods that stabilize your blood sugar, as spikes can cause widespread damage, especially to sensitive nerves.

Don't underestimate the power of movement, even with neuropathy limitations. Find activities that work for you, whether it's short walks, chair yoga, or gentle water exercises. Moving your body boosts circulation (essential for nerve healing) and helps your body combat chronic inflammation.

Finally, remember that stress management isn't a luxury, it's a necessity. Chronic stress triggers the release of hormones that harm both your heart and nerves. Simple mindfulness practices, deep breathing exercises, or even taking a few minutes for a relaxing hobby can make a significant difference when done consistently.

Supplements: Targeted Support for Your Body's Needs

While a healthy diet and lifestyle are foundational, targeted supplements can further enhance your heart and nerve protection. Omega-3 fatty acids, found in fish oil, are superstars when it comes to taming inflammation, benefiting both your blood vessels and those sensitive nerves.

Certain nutrients act like your body's internal blood sugar management team. Magnesium and alpha-lipoic acid are key players, helping to keep blood sugar levels steady and preventing those harmful spikes that contribute to neuropathy.

Lastly, antioxidants like Resveratrol (found in grapes and red wine) and Curcumin (the active compound in turmeric) provide unique protective benefits for your heart and circulatory system, acting as a shield against oxidative damage.

Important Note: Supplements work best when combined with healthy lifestyle changes. Before adding any supplements, always consult with a doctor, especially if you take other medications.

You and Your Heart Health: Making Informed Choices for Nerve Restoration

This chapter isn't about demonizing statins, but about empowering you with knowledge for optimal health decisions. Whether you're currently taking statins or considering them, let's navigate this together.

Working with Your Doctor: A Gradual Approach

If you're on statins, abruptly stopping can be risky. Cholesterol rebound is a concern, so it's crucial to work with your doctor on a safe tapering plan or explore alternative approaches.

Empowering Questions for Your Next Appointment

Don't settle for a passive checkup. Here are some questions to champion your health:

- "What are my specific heart risks, and how does this statin medication address them?"
- "Are there lifestyle modifications I can make to potentially reduce my need for medication?"
- "If I experience new muscle aches, weakness, or difficulty concentrating (brain fog), should I report them right away?"
- "Can we discuss non-statin options for cholesterol management, along with their advantages and disadvantages?"

FREEDOM: A Holistic Approach

Sometimes, statins might be necessary. But even then, the FREEDOM approach remains vital. By addressing inflammation, blood sugar control, and other underlying factors, you're protecting both your heart and nerves, potentially minimizing long-term statin-related side effects. It's about personalized, integrative care, not a one-size-fits-all solution.

Knowledge is Power: Taking Charge of Your Health Journey

This chapter has explored statin function, potential risks, and nourishing alternatives for your whole body. This knowledge equips you, not instills fear. By understanding your medications, you transition from a passive recipient of care to an active participant in your health journey.

Remember, the goal isn't just a lower number on a blood test. True health means thriving nerves, a robust heart, and a life where medications are tools, not a life sentence. Balancing heart health with nerve protection is absolutely achievable. This often involves a combination of smart lifestyle changes, targeted supplements, and carefully considered medications when truly necessary.

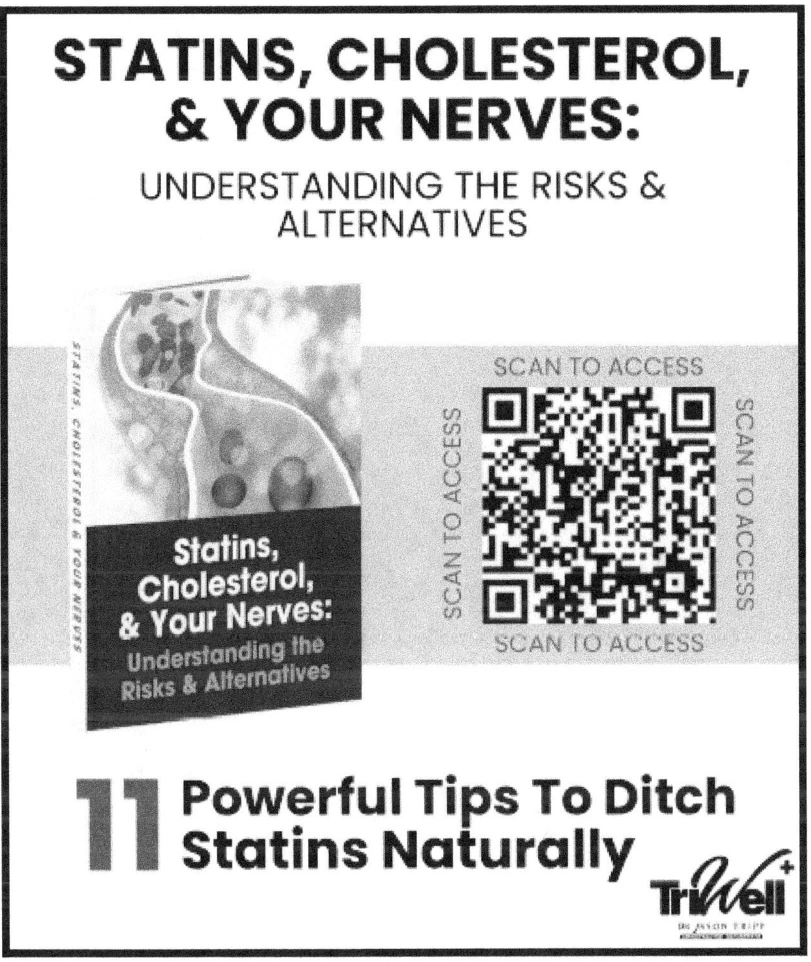

Unlock your Path to Relief Now: Dial (724) 342-2225 to speak with a Neuropathy Care Specialist Today!

9

______

GLUTEN: UNVEILING A POTENTIAL CULPRIT IN NEUROPATHY

Let's delve into gluten, that ever-present protein lurking in many of our foods. If you're battling neuropathy, understanding gluten's potential influence on your health could be a turning point.

Consider how drastically our diets have changed. Gluten isn't just about bread anymore. It's hiding in processed foods, sauces, even medications, leading to constant exposure – especially for those with hidden sensitivities.

The debate surrounding gluten is real. Some doctors dismiss it as a fad, while others are witnessing strong connections between gluten and various health issues, including neuropathy. The truth is, it might not impact everyone equally, but the growing body of research suggesting a link between gluten and nerve damage is undeniable.

Here's the key takeaway: this isn't just about full-blown celiac disease. Gluten sensitivity exists on a spectrum. Even milder sensitivities can trigger significant inflammation throughout your body, and your nerves, unfortunately, aren't immune to those effects.

Gluten: Friend or Foe? Unveiling its Potential Role in Neuropathy

Let's shed light on gluten, a protein naturally found in grains like wheat, rye, and barley. While not inherently bad, it can become problematic for some people, especially those battling neuropathy.

Our modern diet is saturated with gluten, and for some individuals, this constant exposure can be a recipe for trouble. Here's why: People with gluten sensitivity struggle to digest this protein effectively. Imagine undigested gluten-like microscopic velcro lining your gut, irritating and damaging the delicate intestinal lining. This can lead to "leaky gut," a condition where food particles, toxins, and bacteria seep into the bloodstream.

The connection to neuropathy? Leaky gut triggers a cascade of inflammation throughout your body, and chronic inflammation is a major culprit in nerve damage.

Molecular Mimicry: A Stealthy Attack on Your Nerves

Think of your immune system as a highly trained security force. It identifies and eliminates threats like viruses and bacteria. Molecular mimicry is like a villain's clever disguise. In people with gluten sensitivity, the immune system recognizes a resemblance between gluten and components of nerve tissue.

Imagine this: with high inflammation already present, the immune system mistakes gluten for a threat and launches an attack. But here's the tragic twist – it also attacks healthy nerve cells because they bear a similar resemblance to gluten.

This double attack worsens inflammation, creating a vicious cycle that can significantly contribute to neuropathy in some individuals. It emphasizes the critical role of managing inflammation for nerve health, and why identifying potential triggers like gluten is a crucial step in your FREEDOM journey.

Gluten and Neuropathy: The Inflammation Connection

We've explored how gluten sensitivity can trigger widespread inflammation throughout your body. But how does this translate to your experience with neuropathy?

Remember, neuropathy is caused by damaged nerves that struggle to transmit signals properly. Inflammation throws a major wrench into this delicate system. It directly irritates nerves, causing them to misfire and leading to those painful sensations you experience. On top of that, inflammation hinders the body's natural repair mechanisms, further impeding the nerves' ability to heal.

Here are some symptoms that often overlap with gluten sensitivity, making it a potential culprit worth investigating:

- **Digestive Troubles**: Bloating, gas, diarrhea, or constipation are common signs, as your gut is often the first place gluten sensitivity causes problems.
- **Brain Fog**: Difficulty concentrating, fatigue, or mood swings can be linked to gut-related inflammation.
- **Aches and Pains**: Unexplained muscle or joint pain could be a sign of systemic inflammation fueled by gluten.
- **Skin Issues**: Eczema, rashes, and other skin problems are often connected to the gut-inflammation cycle.

It's important to remember that while gluten can be a major contributor to neuropathy for some individuals, it's rarely the sole culprit. Neuropathy is often a complex puzzle with multiple pieces.

Take Jay, for example. He came to us struggling with both neuropathy in his feet and weight problems. His weight had put additional stress on his nerves, further aggravating his neuropathy symptoms. Through the FREEDOM program, we addressed both issues simultaneously. His weight dropped dramatically, and his feet felt "amazingly better," allowing him to sleep peacefully. This case highlights how addressing various factors—not just diet but also lifestyle changes and other underlying health issues—is crucial for achieving lasting relief from neuropathy.

Unveiling Gluten: Beyond the Blood Test and Towards Nerve Restoration

Figuring out if gluten is a culprit in your neuropathy can be frustrating. Standard blood tests often fall short – let's explore why, and discover more reliable ways to find answers.

The Limitations of Celiac Testing

Standard celiac tests target specific antibodies. A positive result is a clear sign of celiac disease. However, what if your immune system reacts differently to gluten? It might involve different antibodies, or an inflammatory response not detectable by a basic blood panel. This means you could still be suffering from gluten sensitivity, even with a negative test result.

The key takeaway: Your body's responses are multifaceted, and a simple blood test might not capture the whole picture. This is why an elimination diet, where you become your own detective, can be a more reliable tool for identifying gluten sensitivity.

The Gold Standard: The Elimination Diet

This strategy involves completely removing gluten from your diet for at least 3-4 weeks, followed by a reintroduction phase. While seemingly straightforward, there are key points to ensure accurate results:

- **Complete Elimination**: Gluten lurks in unexpected places. Meticulous label reading is essential.
- **Track Beyond Neuropathy**: Monitor not just your neuropathy symptoms, but also digestion, energy levels, and any other areas that might improve with gluten removal.
- **Mindful Reintroduction**: Pay close attention to how you feel after reintroducing gluten. A significant symptom flare-up is a strong indicator of sensitivity.

Going Gluten-Free: Embracing the Journey

While ditching gluten can be incredibly beneficial, it's important to be prepared:

- **Nutritional Gaps**: Whole grains offer valuable fiber, iron, and B vitamins. Going gluten-free doesn't mean simply swapping to processed gluten-free alternatives. Focus on incorporating naturally gluten-free whole foods like quinoa, buckwheat, brown rice, legumes, and a vibrant array of fruits and vegetables. This ensures your body receives the essential nutrients for nerve healing.
- **Social Considerations**: Eating out or at friends' places requires a new level of awareness. Plan ahead by checking menus, consider bringing safe options, and advocate for yourself. Finding a supportive community, online or in-person, can make navigating this change much easier.

Not a Standalone Solution

While gluten can be a major trigger for some, it's rarely the sole culprit. Neuropathy is multifaceted. Optimizing blood sugar control, addressing other inflammatory factors, and targeted therapies like those offered in the FREEDOM approach might still be necessary for optimal healing.

Think of going gluten-free as removing a significant roadblock to recovery. It creates the ideal environment for your body and the FREEDOM program to work their magic and support nerve regeneration!

Building on Your Progress: Why FREEDOM is Essential

Removing gluten, if it's a major trigger for you, is a fantastic first step on your journey towards reclaiming your health. But let's explore why the FREEDOM program remains vital, even after making this significant dietary change.

Nerve Healing: A Journey, Not a Destination

Even after eliminating gluten, some nerve damage may still linger. The therapies within the FREEDOM system focus on stimulating the regeneration of those damaged nerves, boosting blood flow to nourish them, and calming any lingering inflammation within the nervous system itself.

A Multifaceted Approach

While gluten sensitivity can be a significant factor, it's not always the sole culprit when it comes to neuropathy. The FREEDOM approach takes a comprehensive view, addressing factors like blood sugar imbalances, stress, and nutritional deficiencies, all of which can significantly impede nerve healing.

Synergy: Where 1 + 1 = 3

Think of removing gluten as clearing away a roadblock, while the FREEDOM therapies act like building a superhighway for optimal nerve communication and repair. When combined, they create a force far more powerful than either approach could be on its own.

Empowered Choices

Understanding how gluten can impact your body is a powerful tool. Regardless of whether it proves to be a major factor for you, this knowledge empowers you to make informed decisions about your health.

Hope and Transformation

By addressing gluten sensitivity (if needed) and utilizing the multifaceted tools of the FREEDOM program, you create the best possible environment for healing and lasting relief from neuropathy. This combination offers a true path to hope and a significant transformation in your health journey.

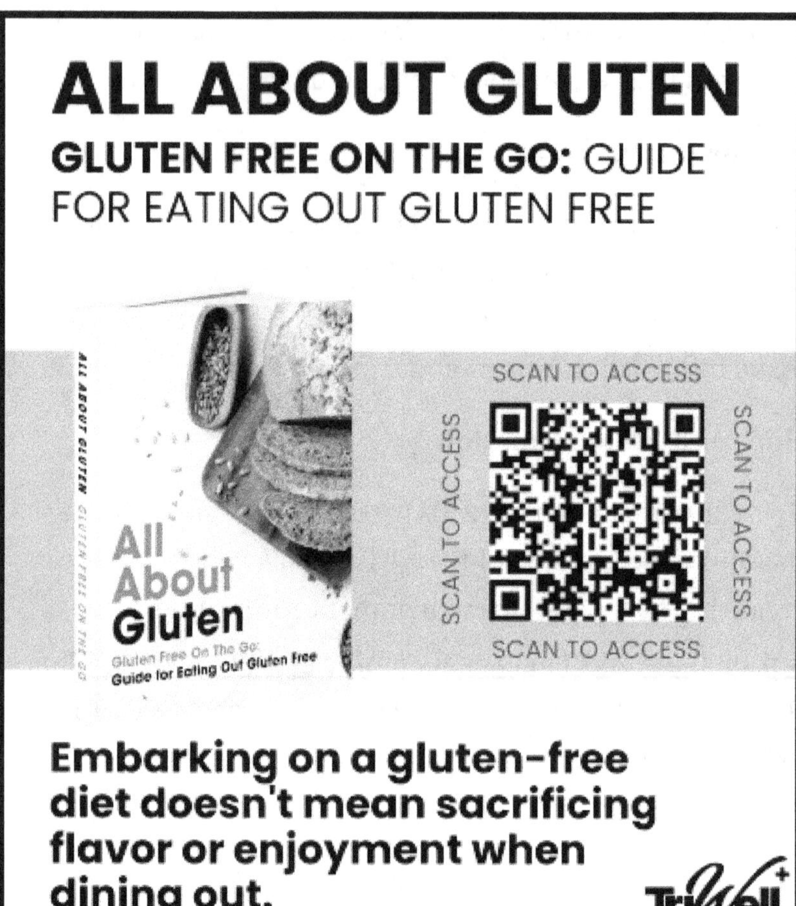

Unlock your Path to Relief Now: Dial (724) 342-2225 to speak with a Neuropathy Care Specialist Today!

10

UNLOCKING NERVE HEALING: RED LIGHT THERAPY, L-ARGININE, & L-CITRULLINE

Red Light Therapy: Shining a Light on Neuropathy Relief

Let's talk about Red Light Therapy (RLT) – think of it as targeted sunlight for deep-tissue healing. RLT devices emit specific wavelengths of red and near-infrared light. Unlike heat lamps, you usually won't feel any warmth during treatment.

Here's the exciting part: Your cells have tiny power plants called mitochondria, responsible for energy production. These specific light wavelengths are absorbed by the mitochondria, giving them a potent energy boost. With more energy, your cells can function better, repair faster, and fight inflammation more effectively.

The science behind RLT isn't just promising – multiple studies show its potential benefits specifically for neuropathy:

- **Reduced Symptoms**: Research suggests RLT can lessen those unpleasant burning, tingling, and other neuropathy sensations, while also improving nerve function and balance.
- **Enhanced Nerve Regeneration**: Lab studies show RLT promotes nerve regrowth after injury, directly benefiting damaged tissues.
- **Improved Blood Flow & Wound Healing**: For diabetics with neuropathy, RLT has demonstrated improved blood flow and wound healing – crucial aspects of managing this complication.

These studies showcase RLT as more than just a fad – it has the potential to significantly improve your experience with neuropathy.

How RLT Can Help You:

- **Taming Inflammation**: Inflammation is a major roadblock to nerve healing. RLT helps calm inflammation in the tissues, creating a more conducive environment for repair.
- **Boosting Circulation**: Healthy blood flow is essential for delivering oxygen and nutrients to

damaged nerves for repair. RLT stimulates blood vessel formation and improves circulation in affected areas.

- **Supporting Nerve Regeneration**: This is perhaps the most exciting benefit. RLT appears to encourage the regrowth of damaged nerve fibers. While not a quick fix, it offers hope for reversing the underlying damage of neuropathy.

Making RLT Work for You:

- **At-Home Devices**: Various RLT devices for home use are available (pads, handheld units, etc.). Look for those used in research studies to ensure quality.
- **In-Office Treatments**: Some chiropractors and physical therapists offer larger, more powerful RLT setups for deeper tissue penetration.
- **Frequency & Duration**: Typically, several treatments per week for several weeks or months are needed to see significant benefits.

Remember, RLT is often most effective when combined with other FREEDOM approaches that address inflammation and promote overall nerve health. By combining these strategies, you can create a powerful path towards lasting relief from neuropathy.

L-Arginine: Nitric Oxide Powerhouse for Nerve Repair

Let's delve into L-Arginine, a small but mighty amino acid that plays a crucial role in nerve health. Think of it as your body's internal construction crew chief, overseeing the building and maintenance of blood vessel highways.

The L-Arginine Advantage

L-Arginine is an amino acid, one of the building blocks of protein. While your body produces some naturally, you can also get it from dietary sources like meat, nuts, and dairy. Here's why it matters for neuropathy: L-Arginine is essential for the production of nitric oxide.

Nitric Oxide: The Blood Flow Regulator

Nitric oxide acts like a traffic controller for your blood vessels. When levels are optimal, it signals vessels to relax and open wider. This isn't just about blood pressure – for nerves, especially those delicate ones in your feet and hands, nitric oxide transforms tiny blood vessels from congested side streets into multi-lane highways.

Imagine your nerves as a remote construction site in desperate need of supplies. Poor circulation means oxygen and vital nutrients trickle in at a snail's pace, hindering repairs. Good blood flow, boosted by nitric oxide, floods the area with the building blocks needed for healing and rebuilding damaged nerves. It's a lifeline for nerve regeneration.

Beyond Blood Flow: A Multifaceted Approach

Nitric oxide's benefits for neuropathy extend far beyond just clearing traffic jams in your blood vessel highways. Remember, neuropathy is a double whammy – nerve damage coupled with inflammation that impedes repair. Nitric oxide tackles both:

- **Taming Inflammation**: Chronic inflammation is like having constant roadblocks around those damaged nerves. Nitric oxide helps quell this inflammatory response, creating a more conducive environment for healing.
- **The Regeneration Spark**: Early research suggests nitric oxide might directly stimulate the process of nerve regrowth. It's like not only delivering supplies to the construction site (your nerves) but also providing the blueprints for rebuilding.

Getting the Right Dose

While a healthy diet rich in L-Arginine (think meat, poultry, fish, and nuts) is beneficial, it might not be enough to significantly impact your nitric oxide levels for nerve healing. Here's what to consider:

- **Food vs. Supplementation**: L-Arginine-rich foods are great, but supplementation, under proper guidance, provides a targeted dose to support nerve repair.

- **Dosage Matters**: There's no one-size-fits-all approach. The right amount for you depends on factors like your overall health and current medications.
- **Safety First**: L-Arginine is generally safe, but talking to your doctor before starting is crucial, especially if you take blood pressure medications, as it can lower blood pressure further. Your doctor can ensure it's the right choice for you and monitor dosage for optimal benefit and safety.

By incorporating L-Arginine, you're giving your body the tools it needs to improve blood flow, reduce inflammation, and potentially promote nerve regeneration – all crucial aspects of the FREEDOM journey.

L-Citrulline: The Supercharged Ally for Nitric Oxide Production

L-Citrulline can be thought of as L-Arginine's more high-achieving cousin. It's another amino acid found in small amounts in foods like watermelon, but its true power for neuropathy lies in supplementation.

Why L-Citrulline? Like L-Arginine, L-Citrulline gets converted into the nitric oxide we discussed earlier, indirectly boosting its production. But here's the exciting part: L-Citrulline may be even more effective at doing so than taking L-Arginine directly!

The Bioavailability Advantage

Imagine your digestive system as a vigilant guard. When you take an L-Arginine supplement, a significant portion gets broken down before reaching its target – the bloodstream. This means much of the potential benefit is lost.

L-Citrulline, on the other hand, bypasses these guards more easily, leading to better absorption. Once absorbed, your body efficiently converts it into L-Arginine. Essentially, L-Citrulline acts like a stealthy way to elevate your L-Arginine levels, maximizing the amount that reaches tissues for healing.

L-Citrulline's Benefits for Neuropathy

Since L-Citrulline supercharges your body's L-Arginine production, its benefits for neuropathy mirror those of L-Arginine:

- **Enhanced Blood Flow**: The increased nitric oxide tells your blood vessels to relax and widen, transforming those narrow passageways leading to damaged nerves into efficient highways. This translates to improved delivery of oxygen and essential nutrients for repair.
- **Reduced Pain**: L-Citrulline offers a double benefit

for pain relief. Improved blood flow eases burning and tingling sensations, while it also tackles chronic inflammation, a known amplifier of nerve pain.

- **Potential for Regeneration**: Early research suggests L-Citrulline might go beyond just boosting circulation. There's evidence it may assist in nerve regeneration itself, not just delivering building materials but also potentially helping create a more efficient "construction crew" for nerve repair.

Dosage and Safety: As always, individual needs dictate the optimal dosage. Let's discuss what's right for you and ensure it doesn't interact with any medications you're currently taking.

By incorporating L-Citrulline, you're providing your body with a powerful tool to increase nitric oxide production, improve blood flow, reduce inflammation, and potentially promote nerve regeneration – all crucial aspects of your FREEDOM journey.

The FREEDOM Advantage: Synergy and Natural Healing

The power of FREEDOM lies in synergy – combining tools that amplify each other's effects. This is where Red Light Therapy, L-Arginine, and L-Citrulline become a truly powerful trio against neuropathy.

A Multifaceted Approach

Imagine each tool tackling neuropathy from a unique angle:

- Red Light Therapy: Works on a cellular level, reducing inflammation and promoting nerve regeneration.
- L-Arginine & L-Citrulline: Enhance blood flow, ensuring crucial oxygen and nutrients reach damaged nerves.

The result? Rather than isolated benefits, they work together to create the ideal environment for nerve healing. It's a symphony of effects, greater than the sum of its parts.

The Natural Path to Relief

Compared to traditional neuropathy treatments that often mask symptoms or come with side effects, these approaches leverage your body's inherent healing mechanisms. This translates to a generally safer and gentler path toward lasting relief.

A word of caution: Even though these are natural therapies, discussing them with your doctor, chiropractor, or qualified healthcare professional is still crucial. We can provide personalized dosing recommendations and ensure no conflicts with medications you're taking.

The Takeaway: Empowering Your Body to Heal

We've explored how Red Light Therapy, L-Arginine, and L-Citrulline can be valuable allies in your fight against neuropathy. Remember, these are potent tools that work with your body's natural healing potential. They reduce inflammation, improve blood flow, and may even directly support nerve regeneration.

While not instant fixes, these therapies empower you to take an active role in your health. Instead of simply masking symptoms, you're addressing the underlying factors that impede healing. They create the optimal environment for your body to repair and rebuild – the true path to freedom from the grip of neuropathy.

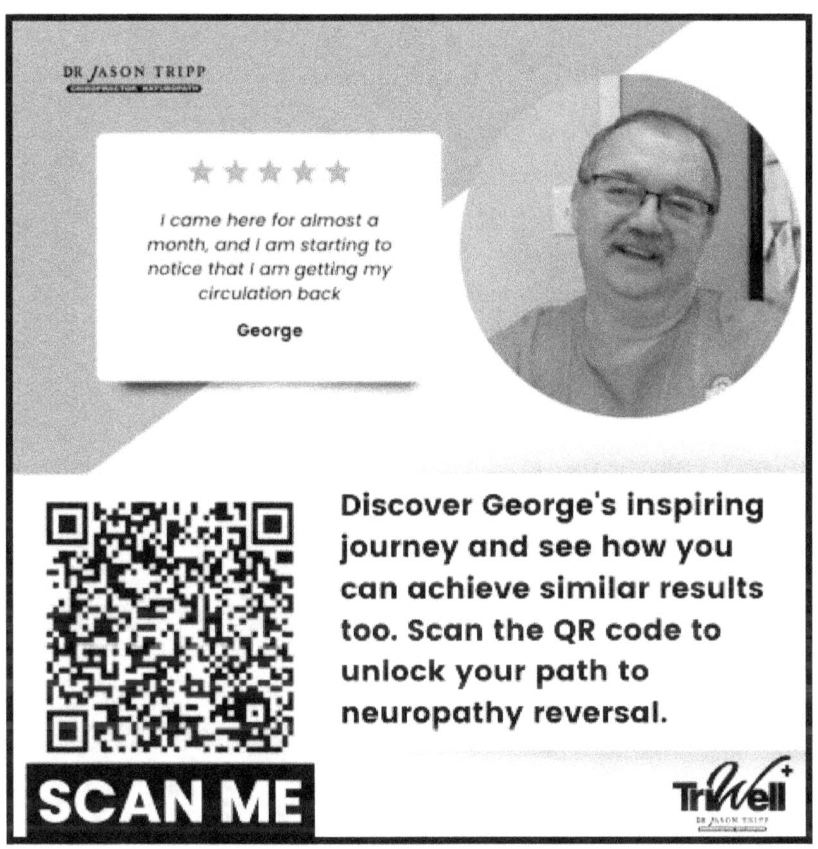

Unlock your Path to Relief Now: Dial (724) 342-2225 to speak with a Neuropathy Care Specialist Today!

11

OPIOIDS: WHY WE LOOK FOR ALTERNATIVE SOLUTIONS

As we explore conquering neuropathy, it's impossible to ignore the other epidemic impacting millions: opioid addiction. Let's be clear – this isn't about blaming those struggling with opioids, but rather highlighting the dangers, especially for those suffering from chronic pain like neuropathy.

The statistics are alarming. Opioid overdose deaths have risen dramatically in recent years, with chronic pain as a major contributing factor. According to the Centers for Disease Control and Prevention (CDC), more than 1 million people have died since 1999 from a drug overdose, and more than 75% of drug overdose deaths involved an opioid. It's a vicious cycle – someone in constant agony seeks medication for relief, often unaware of the slippery slope it can be.

Neuropathy creates a perfect storm for opioid vulnerability. The unrelenting burning, tingling, or electric shock sensations can push even the most resilient person to a breaking point. In that moment of desperation, powerful painkillers might seem like the only answer.

While there may be rare cases where short-term opioid use is necessary under strict medical supervision, it's crucial to understand the significant risks involved. What feels like a lifeline initially can quickly become a dangerous trap. FREEDOM offers a different approach, focusing on addressing the root causes of neuropathy pain and promoting natural healing mechanisms within your body.

Opioids: Masking Pain, Not Healing Nerves

Opioids present a significant challenge in the fight against neuropathy. While they may offer a false sense of relief, they fail to address the root cause of the problem – nerve damage. Let's delve into why this makes them an unsuitable long-term solution for neuropathy.

Turning Down the Volume, Not Stopping the Fire

Imagine neuropathy as a burning building. Opioids act like a faulty fire alarm silencer – they block the pain signals reaching your brain, essentially muting the alarm. While you might feel a sense of relief, the fire itself – the damaged nerves – continues to rage on unabated. The underlying issue remains unresolved.

The Tolerance Trap

Our bodies are remarkably adaptable. Over time, with continued opioid use, they build a tolerance. The initial dose that provided relief may no longer be effective. This triggers a dangerous cycle. To chase that numbing effect, people often escalate their dosage, taking more and more pills. The focus shifts from managing pain to simply avoiding withdrawal symptoms.

The FREEDOM approach takes a different path. We focus on addressing the underlying causes of neuropathy pain and promoting natural healing mechanisms within your body. This holistic approach aims to not just quiet the alarm, but to extinguish the fire altogether.

The Dark Side of Opioids: Why They Aren't the Answer for Neuropathy

Opioids for neuropathy come with a hefty price tag, far exceeding the risk of addiction. Even when taken as prescribed, side effects can significantly worsen your neuropathy experience.

Beyond Addiction: A Multitude of Issues

- **Digestive Distress**: Opioids often cause severe constipation, leading to a domino effect of problems. Straining can aggravate existing issues like hemorrhoids or hernias, while backed-up toxins worsen inflammation, a major roadblock to nerve healing.

- **Brain Fog**: Forget occasional forgetfulness. Opioids can induce a persistent mental fog that compounds the cognitive challenges often associated with neuropathy. Everyday tasks become difficult, work suffers, and connecting with loved ones becomes a struggle.

- **Hormonal Havoc**: Opioids disrupt your delicate hormonal balance, impacting sleep (making neuropathy pain harder to manage), mood (leading to low feelings and irritability), and metabolism (affecting weight and energy levels). These changes chip away at your well-being, making fighting neuropathy even more uphill.

Opioids and Worsening Neuropathy: A Catch-22

Emerging research suggests a concerning link between opioids and long-term nerve damage – exactly what we're trying to avoid with neuropathy treatment. Here's why exploring alternative solutions is crucial.

Potential Damage Mechanisms: While research is ongoing, several theories exist:

- Opioids may elevate inflammation and oxidative

stress, further harming already compromised nerves.

- They might directly damage sensory receptors within the nerves themselves.
- By suppressing natural pain signals, they could delay seeking interventions that could actually heal the neuropathy.

A Crippling Cycle: How Opioids Trap You

The opioid trap for neuropathy patients is particularly insidious. Let's break down a potential scenario:

1. **Desperation for Relief**: You begin taking opioids, initially finding pain relief.
2. **Tolerance and Return of Pain**: Over time, your body builds tolerance, with those painful symptoms creeping back.
3. **The Fallacy of "More is Better"**: Thinking a higher dose equals better relief, you (or sometimes even your doctor) unconsciously escalate the dosage. This offers temporary relief but silently worsens the underlying neuropathy.
4. **Repeat and Escalate**: More pain necessitates an even higher dose, perpetuating the cycle.

Opioids cut off pain perception, creating the illusion of solving the problem. But the nerve damage continues, making you believe you need the medication even more. The drug transforms from a pain management tool to the primary driver of your pain.

Breaking free from this cycle is incredibly difficult due to physical dependence. That's why addressing neuropathy at its root and exploring safer alternatives is crucial before the addiction risk escalates. FREEDOM focuses on healing the underlying causes of neuropathy pain, empowering your body to heal naturally.

Escaping the Opioid Cycle: Hope and Practical Steps for Nerve Restoration

Breaking free from opioid dependence for neuropathy pain is undeniably challenging, but it's absolutely achievable. Let's explore this message of hope alongside practical steps and support systems to guide you toward success.

There's No Shame in Seeking Help

Opioid addiction can happen to anyone grappling with relentless pain. Recognizing the need for help is a powerful first step. You're not alone; there are resources readily available to support you on your journey to freedom.

Safe Tapering: A Must-Have

Quitting opioids abruptly (cold turkey) is incredibly

dangerous and leads to severe withdrawal symptoms. These can include:

- Intense muscle aches and flu-like symptoms
- Anxiety, restlessness, and insomnia
- Digestive issues (nausea, diarrhea, vomiting)
- Changes in blood pressure and heart rate

The severity varies, but the experience is undeniably difficult. This is why attempting to quit without medical supervision is a risky proposition. It often leads to relapse simply to find relief, even for those who desperately want to break free.

An addiction medicine specialist can design a slow, personalized tapering plan based on your individual dosage and history. This minimizes withdrawal symptoms, making them more manageable. While still challenging, the process becomes more tolerable, increasing your chances of lasting success.

The Root of the Problem

The key to lasting freedom from opioids lies in addressing the root cause of pain – your neuropathy itself. Instead of simply numbing the symptoms, the FREEDOM approach focuses on healing those damaged nerves. As the pain naturally lessens and your function improves, dependence on medication decreases organically. This offers a sustainable path towards a pain-free future, not just a temporary fix.

Beyond Tapering: Building a Support System

Breaking free from opioids goes beyond just the medication. Here are some additional strategies for lasting success:

- **Therapy**: Talking to a therapist can help you understand and manage the emotional aspects of pain and addiction.
- **Support Groups**: Connecting with others who share your struggles can provide invaluable encouragement and accountability.
- **Pain Management Techniques**: Techniques like mindfulness meditation, acupuncture, and exercise can empower you to cope with pain in a healthier way.

Remember, you are not alone in this fight. With the right support system, a focus on FREEDOM, and a safe tapering plan, you can break free from the cycle of opioid dependence and reclaim your life from chronic pain.

Breaking the Cycle: Early Action and Open Communication Are Key

Let's shift our focus to preventing the devastating opioid cycle altogether. The key lies in the proactive management of neuropathy and fostering open communication with your healthcare team.

The longer neuropathy pain goes unaddressed, the greater the risk of turning to opioids in a desperate search for relief. Seeking FREEDOM care as soon as possible is vital. When pain is effectively managed from the outset, the temptation of quick fixes with potentially dangerous side effects significantly diminishes.

Honesty is Key: Be upfront with your doctor about the severity of your neuropathy pain, even if you fear judgment. Don't downplay your suffering! Open communication allows us to explore safer and more effective alternatives early on – targeted therapies, specific exercises, and non-opioid pain management strategies tailored to your unique needs.

While battling opioid addiction requires immense courage, there is immense hope. Addiction does not define you, and with the right support, it can be overcome.

A Path to True Healing

It's time to choose a different path – one that leads to genuine healing, not just masked pain. Whether you're concerned about yourself or a loved one, FREEDOM offers a powerful alternative. True healing doesn't just address the physical symptoms of neuropathy – it protects your overall well-being and empowers you to reclaim control over your life.

Neuropathy Reversed: Dave's Miracle

"I had neuropathy due to diabetes in both of my feet. The pain had become excruciating. All doctors could do is prescribe pills to manage the pain. Then, I met Dr. Tripp. He has been able to reverse the nerve damage, relieve the pain, and restore the sense of touch. This is a man who is doing God's own work—a miracle." - Dave M.

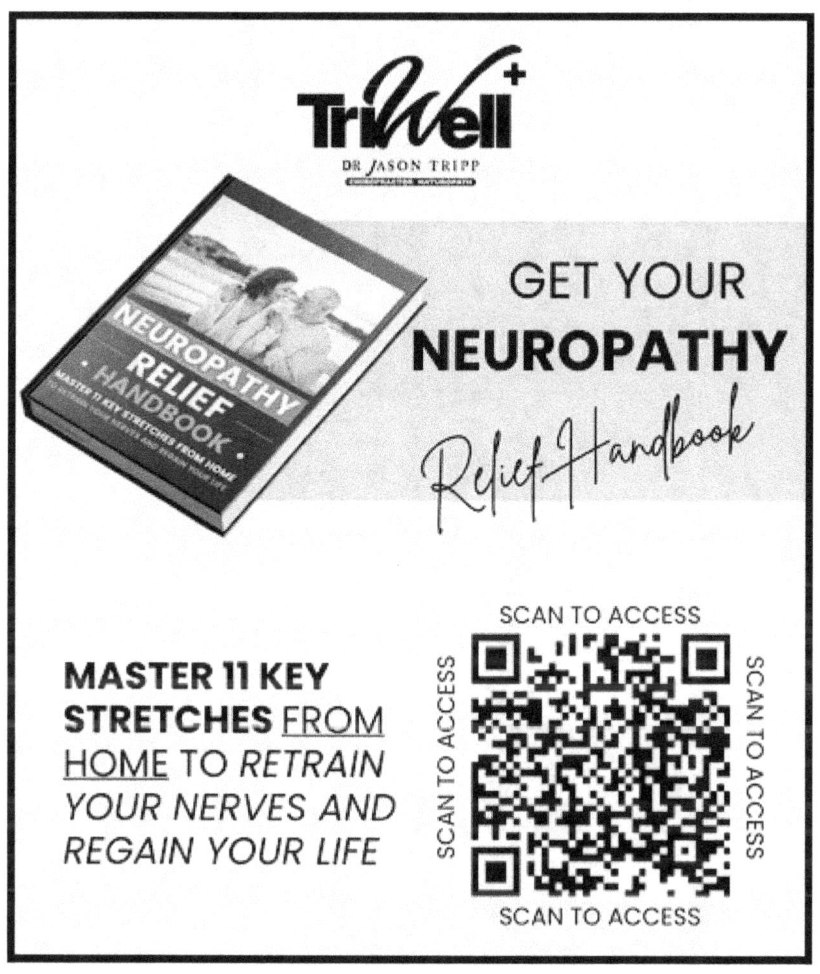

Unlock your Path to Relief Now: Dial (724) 342-2225 to speak with a Neuropathy Care Specialist Today!

12

EMBARK ON THE FREEDOM JOURNEY: RECLAIM YOUR HEALTH, YOUR LIFE

The other day, Rose walked into my office with a bounce in her step and a grin that could outshine the sun. "My feet ain't sizzling anymore, Doc!" she exclaimed, her voice brimming with a joy that echoed the victory she'd achieved over her neuropathy. Three weeks ago, that same walk had been a laborious endeavor, each step a painful reminder of the nerve damage that had been stealing her freedom. She'd described her feet as constantly "sizzling," a feeling so intense it made even the simplest tasks a monumental effort.

Seeing Rose transform from a woman burdened by pain and limitations to one radiating hope and vitality is the very reason I do what I do. It's a testament to the power of the FREEDOM neuropathy method, a holistic approach designed to help individuals like Rose reclaim their health and rediscover the joy of living.

Your journey to overcome neuropathy and regain your quality of life begins with a single, decisive step – a commitment to the FREEDOM neuropathy method. This holistic approach, rooted in scientific principles and personalized care, offers a powerful pathway to managing neuropathy and transforming your overall health.

The FREEDOM journey requires dedication, a willingness to adopt healthy lifestyle changes, and an unwavering belief in your ability to heal. When you commit to this program, you are taking control of your health and beginning a journey toward a thriving and flourishing you.

Take the First Step: Come to our Seminar

Congratulations on making it this far in the book! Your dedication to reversing your neuropathy is truly inspiring. You now understand the complexities of this condition, the pitfalls of quick fixes, and the potential for true healing through the FREEDOM Method. But knowledge without action is like a seed unplanted - it holds potential but bears no fruit. Are you ready to cultivate that potential and see real change in your life?

The first step towards that transformation is joining me, Dr. Jason Tripp, for a LIVE, in-person seminar. This is your opportunity to dive deeper into the FREEDOM neuropathy method, get personalized insights, and discover if you're a good candidate to reverse your neuropathy naturally without drugs or surgery. This seminar will provide you with valuable information, answer your questions, and empower you to make an informed decision about your health. Click HERE to Reserve Your Seat

More FREEDOM Success Stories

Elaine's Story: How Three Visits Changed Her Life

"I was always in pain because of my numb foot, but after three visits with Dr. Tripp, I was actually able to ride the motorcycle all over Florida on vacation, and I was able to walk all over Disney World with no pain. And when I came back, I couldn't believe how great I felt after vacation."

Linda's Leap: From Neuropathy to High Heels

"I've been coming to Tripp Chiropractic & Nutrition for three months, and now I feel great. I'm able to wear high-heeled shoes, and when I'm driving, I can feel the gas pedal under me. So it's been magnificent. Doctor Tripp is my hero. The staff is great, and I feel great!"

Sharon's Journey: From Neuropathy to Nurtured Spirits

"Tripp Chiropractic & Nutrition has really helped me. The staff really takes the time to listen to you. My husband sees that I'm happy like now, I feel more relaxed. The neuropathy program has lifted my spirit because my neuropathy in my feet was making me a little depressed. But now I'm feeling good, and I have more energy. Dr. Tripp has really made a difference because he cares, his team cares, and I am glad that I am started on this journey."

Margaret's Triumph: From Frozen Hands to Freedom

"I came up to Tripp Chiropractic & Nutrition, and I could hardly walk. My left side was always messed up. My hands and everything would freeze up. I've been coming up to see him for over a year now, and I'm really happy. I would recommend Dr. Tripp to anybody who has neuropathy."

Visualize Your Success

As you start on a course of action, take time to visualize the positive changes you hope to achieve. Envision yourself managing your neuropathy symptoms effectively, engaging in activities you once enjoyed, and living a life filled with vitality and zest. Your mental focus and unwavering belief in your ability to heal will be powerful motivators throughout your FREEDOM journey.

Don't let neuropathy hold you back from living your best life. The FREEDOM method is more than just a treatment; it's a transformation. It's a way to reclaim your health, your vitality, and your freedom.

Do you want to wake up every morning feeling energized and pain-free? Do you want to enjoy your favorite activities without worrying about your nerves? Do you want to feel confident and optimistic about your future? If you answered yes, then you are ready for the FREEDOM method.

This is your chance to embrace the journey, embrace the commitment, and embrace the possibility of becoming healthier and happier. Take action now, and I look forward to meeting you soon.

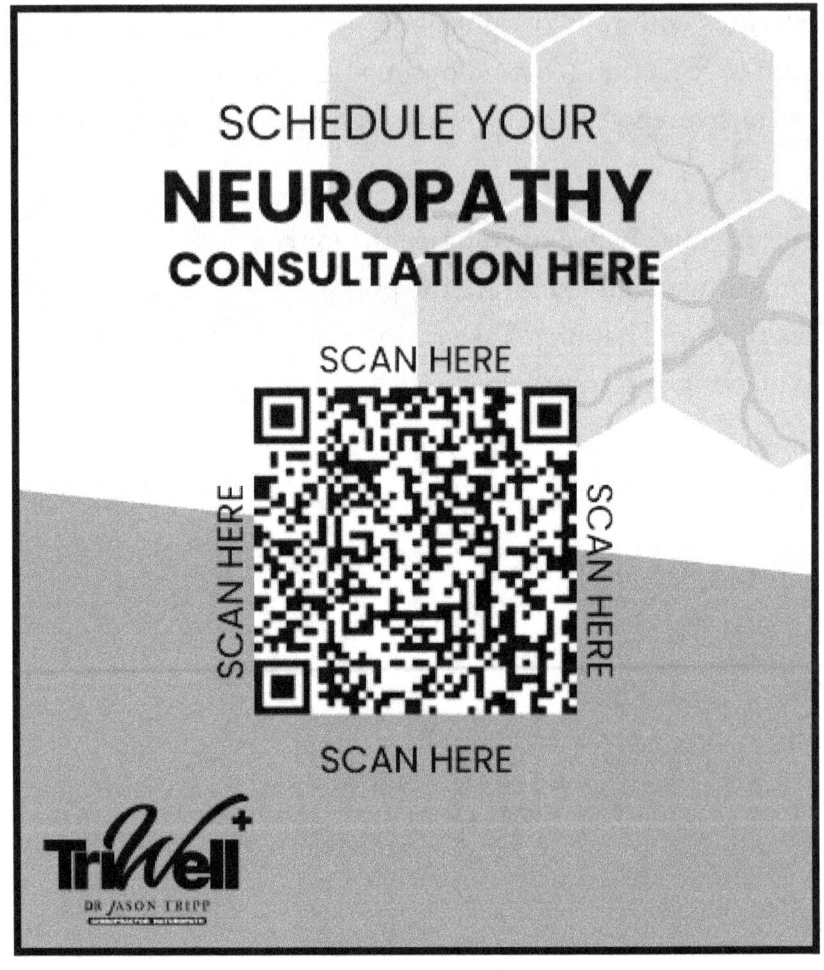

Unlock your Path to Relief Now: Dial (724) 342-2225 to speak with a Neuropathy Care Specialist Today!

Not in Sharon or surrounding cities? Watch our free masterclass to learn more about FREEDOM.

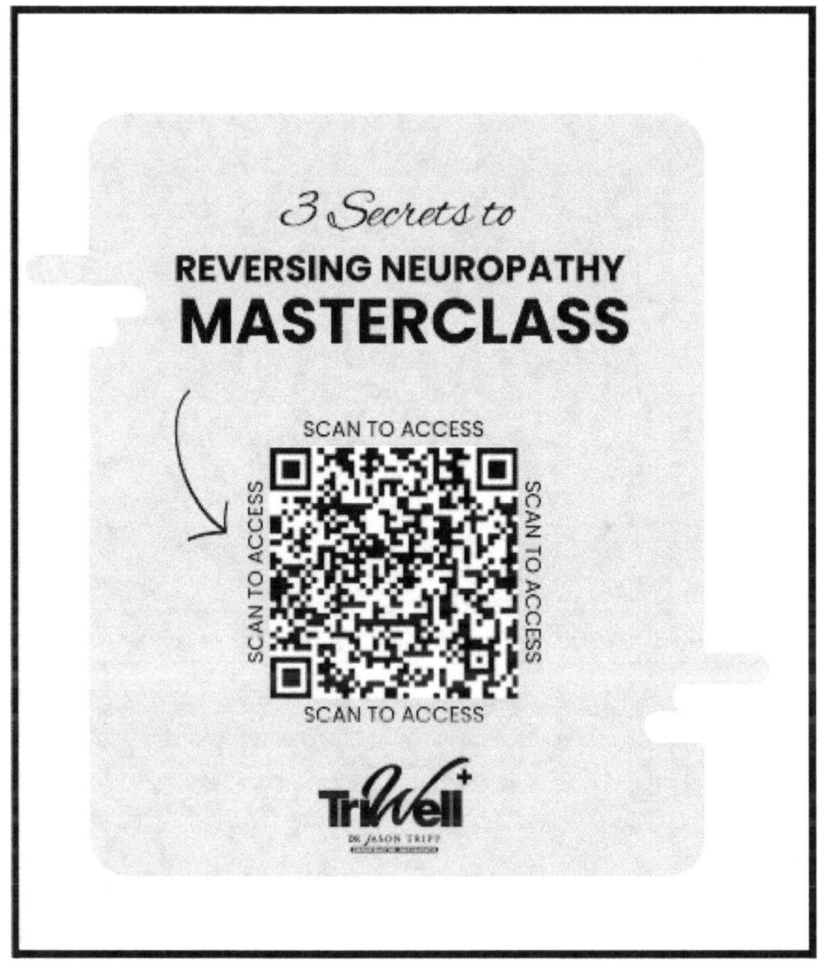

Unlock your Path to Relief Now: Dial (724) 342-2225 to speak with a Neuropathy Care Specialist Today!

SOURCES

- McKinley-Barnard et al. Combined L-citrulline and glutathione supplementation increases the concentration of markers indicative of nitric oxide synthesis. Journal of the International Society of Sports Nutrition (2015) 12:27.
- Kochman AB, Carnegie DE, Burke TJ. Symptomatic Reversal of Peripheral Neuropathy in
- Patients with Diabetes. Journal of the American Podiatric Medical Association. 2002;92:125-130.
- Prendergast JJ, Miranda G, Sanchez M. Improvement of Sensory Impairment in Patients with Peripheral Neuropathy. Endocrine Practice. 2004;10:24-30.
- Leonard DR, Farooqi MH, Myers S. Restoration of Sensation, Reduced Pain, and Improved Balance in Subjects with Diabetic Peripheral Neuropathy; A Randomized, Double Blind, Placebo Controlled Study. Diabetes Care. 2004;27:168-172.
- Kochman AB. Monochromatic Infrared Photo Energy and Physical Therapy for Peripheral Neuropathy: Influence on Sensation, Balance and Falls. Journal of Geriatric Physical Therapy. 2004;27:16-19.
- Harkless L, DeLellis S, Burke TJ. Improved Foot Sensitivity and Pain Reduction in Patients with Peripheral Neuropathy after Treatment with Monochromatic Infrared Photo Energy-MIRE. Journal of Diabetes and Its Complications. 2006;20(2):81-87.
- Ammar, T. Monochromatic Infrared Photo Energy in Diabetic Peripheral Neuropathy. International Scholarly Research Network (ISRN) Rehabilitation. 2012; Article ID 484307.
- Stanley Paul, Yuanlong liu, Robert McAlister The efficacy of monochromatic infrared photo-thermal energy therapy in

rehabilitation: A pilot study report. Indian Journal of Physiotherapy and Occupational Therapy. January –March 2010, Vol.4, No.1

- Chen, Y et al. Extracorporeal shock wave therapy effectively prevented diabetic neuropathy. American Journal Transl Res 2015;7(12):2543-2560.
- Hausner T, Nógrádi A. The Use of Shock Waves in Peripheral Nerve Regeneration: New Perspectives? International Review of Neurobiology, 2013. Volume 109
- Schuh, C. M. A. P., Hercher, D., Stainer, M., Hopf, R., Teuschl, A. H., Schmidhammer, R., & Redl, H. Extracorporeal shockwave treatment: A novel tool to improve Schwann cell isolation and culture. Cytotherapy 2016, 18(6), 760–770.
- Hausner, T. et al. Improved rate of peripheral nerve regeneration induced by extracorporeal shock wave treatment in the rat. Experimental Neurology 2012, 236(2), 363–370.

www.ingramcontent.com/pod-product-compliance
Lightning Source LLC
Chambersburg PA
CBHW071433130726
47997CB00006B/2072